世界の
インパクトファクターを決める
トムソン・ロイター社が
選出

エンドのための重要20キーワード ベスト240論文

講演や雑誌でよく見る、あの分類および文献

監修 須田英明　著者 金子友厚／伊藤崇史／山本信一

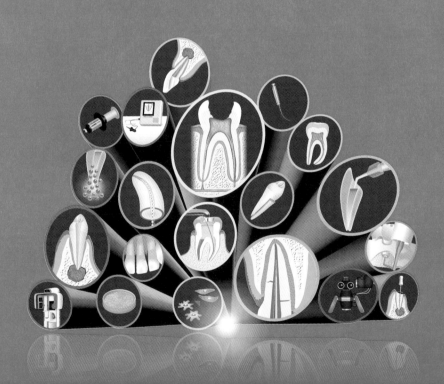

クインテッセンス出版株式会社　2015

Tokyo, Berlin, Chicago, London, Paris, Barcelona, Istanbul, Milano, São Paulo, Moscow, Prague, Warsaw, Delhi, Bucharest, and Singapore

序文

歯内療法を学ぶ方法・機会は数多い。教科書、参考書、学術雑誌、オンラインジャーナル、学術大会、講演会、講習会、スタディグループ、DVD、ウェブサイトなど、枚挙にいとまがない。今やわれわれは溢れんばかりの歯内療法関連の情報を、いつでも簡単に入手できるようになった。他方、歯内療法に携わる者は、それらの多量・多彩な情報を整理して体系化しなければ、多様な歯内療法症例を現実に対応できない。ベストの治療選択肢はどれか？　その理論的・臨床的裏付けはあるのか？　ときには相反する情報に遭遇することもある。臨床現場において、治療に迷いが生じることは少なくない。

本書は、従来にはみられなかった斬新な手法で、読者へ歯内療法関連情報を提供することを試みている。すなわち、トムソン・ロイター社によって抽出された、歯内療法における20の最新キーワードについて、被引用数がもっとも多い12の論文をそれぞれ紹介し、解説を加えている。いい換えれば、現代の歯内療法に大きな影響を及ぼしている重要論文を速習できるよう、配慮がなされている。選ばれた20のキーワードは、歯髄炎、根尖病変、垂直性歯根破折、根管長測定器、あるいはNi-Ti製ロータリーファイルなど、現代の歯内療法における重要項目ばかりである。

独創的な企画で刊行された本書が、読者にどのような評価を受けるかは予測できない。しかし、現場で困難な歯内療法症例に直面して岐路に立たされることの多い臨床医や、新しい理論・技術・器材の開発に日頃努力している研究者にとって、自身の知識を整理するのに大いに役立つことは確かである。また、スタディグループや大学・企業等の研究機関における歯内療法教材としての利用価値は高いと思われる。

本書の完成には、金子友厚博士(新潟大学大学院医歯学総合研究科・口腔健康科学講座・う蝕学分野)が尽力された。かつて同氏は私の主宰する教室に所属していたが、氏の学術論文作成および論文査読能力は抜群である。ここに心より敬意を表し、本書の完成を支えた吉田敏明氏(クインテッセンス出版株式会社、ザ・クインテッセンス編集部)とともに発刊をお祝い申し上げる次第である。

むすびに、本書が契機・推進エンジンとなって、わが国の歯内療法の知識・技術がさらに向上することを願うものである。

2015年9月
東京医科歯科大学名誉教授
須田英明

著者略歴

金子友厚（Kaneko Tomoatsu）

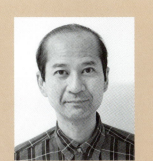

平成 8 年　東京医科歯科大学・歯学部卒
平成12年　東京医科歯科大学・大学院・歯科保存学系修了
平成14年　東京医科歯科大学大学院・医歯学総合研究科・歯髄生物学分野・助手
平成14年　日本歯科保存学会奨励賞
平成16年～平成18年　米国ミシガン大学 Department of Cariology, Restorative Sciences, and Endodontics; Postdoctoral research fellow（Teaching Staff 兼任）
平成21年　日本歯科保存学会学術賞
平成21年～現在　Journal of Tissue Engineering Editorial Board
平成22年～現在　新潟大学医歯学総合病院・歯の診療科（う蝕学分野）・助教
平成26年～現在　Journal of Dental Research Editorial Board
平成26年　日本歯内療法学会ワカイ賞

伊藤崇史（Ito Takafumi）

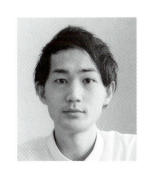

平成23年　新潟大学・歯学部卒
平成23年～平成24年　新潟大学医歯学総合病院・歯科総合診療部
平成24年～現在　新潟大学大学院医歯学総合研究科・う蝕顎分野
平成27年～現在　新潟大学医歯学総合病院医療連携口腔管理チーム(歯内療法担当)

山本信一（Yamamoto Shinichi）

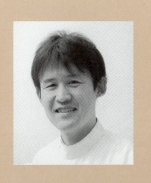

平成 7 年　新潟大学・歯学部卒
平成 7 年～平成19年　大阪府内の医療法人に勤務
平成19年～現在　宝塚市にて山本歯科クリニックを開院

Contents

序文 ... 2
本書の読み方 ... 6
本書を読む前に知っておくべきキーワード ... 8

重要キーワード20 ... 9

1. Pulpitis ... 10
2. Periapical lesion ... 18
3. Vertical root fracture ... 25
4. Apex locators ... 33
5. Rotary nickel-titanium instruments ... 41
6. Curved root canals ... 48
7. Root canal transportation ... 55
8. Endodontic irrigation ... 62
9. Sodium hypochlorite ... 70
10. EDTA ... 77
11. Calcium hydroxide ... 84
12. Root canal condensation ... 91
13. Microleakage ... 99
14. Endodontic microsurgery ... 106
15. Endodontic treatment outcomes ... 114

- 16. Mineral trioxide aggregate — 121
- 17. Cone-beam computed tomography — 128
- 18. Pulp revascularization — 135
- 19. Dental pulp tissue engineering — 143
- 20. Dental pulp cells — 151

分類 — 159

1. 根管形態の分類 — 160
2. イスムス形態の分類 — 162
3. 上顎第一大臼歯近心頰側根 — 164
4. 上顎第一大臼歯近心舌側根管の探知 — 165
5. 下顎大臼歯近心中央根管について — 166
6. 受動的超音波洗浄法 — 167
7. 臨床所見に基づく根尖性歯周組織疾患の分類 — 168
8. 根尖部エックス線透過像と歯内療法の成功率 — 169
9. 外傷歯破折の分類 — 170
10. 亀裂歯の分類 — 171
11. 根尖外科手術1年後のエックス線写真所見 — 172
12. 歯内療法における微生物 — 173
13. 細菌関連物質 — 174
14. 幹細胞のタンパクおよび遺伝子のプロフィール — 175

本書の見方

概要
インパクトファクターの決定やノーベル賞の受賞者予測で知られるトムソン・ロイターの Web of Science® を利用し、エンド関連の講演や発表および治療において重要な 20 キーワードで論文検索を行った。
　本書は、検索結果を被引用件数順に並び替え、上位 12 件を列記した。さらに 12 論文を編集委員会にて吟味し、キーワードに照らして臨床における関連性・重要性・有益性の高い 4〜5 論文についての抄録を掲載した。
　加えて学会や講演会、雑誌などに頻回登場し、必読と思われる分類や論文を、可及的に原著論文を基に添付した。

用語解説

① 検索キーワード
Web of Science® 上にて検索に用いたキーワード。カテゴリーを選択（タイトルもしくはトピック）して検索する。"AND" でキーワードの重複論文が、"OR" でいずれかに該当する論文が、また "NOT" でそのキーワードを含まない論文が選択される。

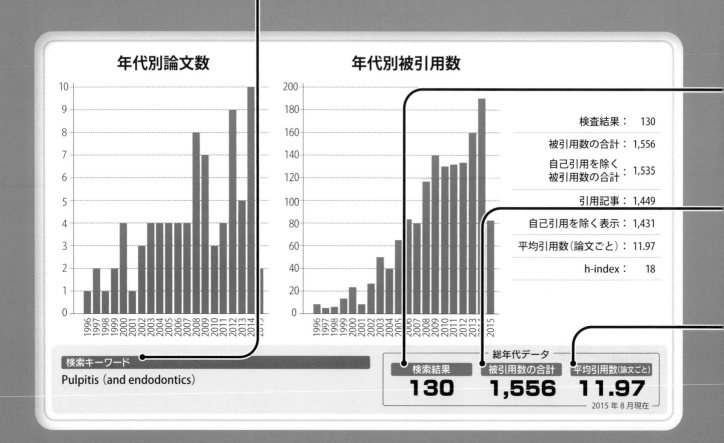

トムソン・ロイターが選んだベスト**12**論文

	タイトル・和訳	2011年	2012年	2013年	2014年	合計引用数
引用数 **1位**	Love RM, Jenkinson HF. Invasion of dentinal tubules by oral bacteria. Crit Rev Oral Biol Med 2002；13(2)：171-183. 口腔内細菌による象牙細管の浸潤 **本項に和訳あり**	10	15	19	23	165
引用数 **2位**	Nakashima M, Akamine A. The application of tissue engineering to regeneration of pulp and dentin in endodontics. J Endod 2005；31(10)：711-718. 歯内療法における歯髄および象牙質を再生するための組織工学の応用 **本項に和訳あり**	17	11	16	15	122
引用数 **3位**	Weiger R, Hitzler S, Hermle G, Löst C. Periapical status, quality of root canal fillings and estimated endodontic treatment needs in urban an German population. Endod Dent Traumatol 1997；13(2)：69-74. ドイツ都市部の住民における根尖周囲の状態、根管充填の質、および推定される根管治療ニーズ量 **本項に和訳あり**	10	8	7	4	8
引用数 **4位**	Eriksen HM. Endodontology-epidemiologic considerations. Traumatol 1991；7(5)：189-195. 歯内療法学―疫学的検討 **本項に和訳あり**					60
引用数 **5位**	...eid TM, Pearson GJ. Microbiological evaluation of ...tion in endodontics (an *in vivo* study). Br Dent J 歯内療法における光殺菌に関する微生物学的評価（*in vivo* での研究） **本項に和訳あり**	11	5	4	4	50
引用数 **6位**	... a review. J Endod 2000；26(3)：175-	1	5	3	6	44

② 検索結果
キーワードを基に検索された総論文数

③ 被引用数の合計
②で検索された総論文の被引用数の合計

④ 平均引用数（論文ごと）
該当キーワードにおける1論文あたりの平均引用数（③を②で割ったもの）

⑤ 合計引用数
各論文が発表されてから2015年8月までにおける被引用数の合計

1 Pulpitis

本書を読む前に知っておくべきキーワード

トムソン・ロイターとは？

世界の約 11,000 の学術誌に掲載された論文をデータベース化して提供し、3,800以上の研究機関が利用している。学術誌の質の指標となる「インパクトファクター」の発案や毎年のノーベル賞受賞者の予測でも知られる。

(朝日新聞より引用・改変)

インパクトファクターとは？

インパクトファクター（文献引用影響率）とは、特定のジャーナル（学術雑誌）に掲載された論文が特定の年または期間内にどれくらい頻繁に引用されたかを平均値で示す尺度である。これはトムソン・ロイターの Journal Citation Reports® (JCR®) が備えている評価ツールの1つである。

毎年 JCR® が公開する特定のジャーナルのインパクトファクターは、対象年における被引用回数を、対象年に先立つ2年間にそのジャーナルが掲載した論文の総数で割ることによって計算する。

インパクトファクターを保持することがジャーナルのステータスであるとともに、インパクトファクターが高いほどジャーナルの価値が高いとされる。（例：Nature、The New England Journal of Medicine）

(トムソン・ロイターHPより引用・改変)

$$\text{インパクトファクター} = \frac{\text{対象年にそのジャーナルが掲載した論文が引用された回数}}{\text{対象年に先立つ2年間にそのジャーナルが掲載した論文の総数}}$$

重要キーワード20

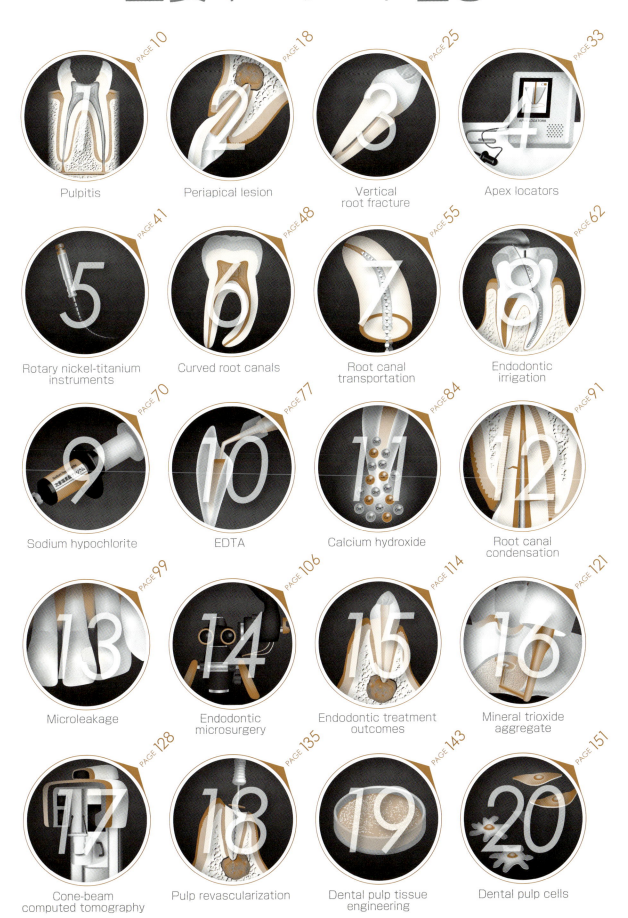

PAGE 10 — 1. Pulpitis
PAGE 18 — 2. Periapical lesion
PAGE 25 — 3. Vertical root fracture
PAGE 33 — 4. Apex locators
PAGE 41 — 5. Rotary nickel-titanium instruments
PAGE 48 — 6. Curved root canals
PAGE 55 — 7. Root canal transportation
PAGE 62 — 8. Endodontic irrigation
PAGE 70 — 9. Sodium hypochlorite
PAGE 77 — 10. EDTA
PAGE 84 — 11. Calcium hydroxide
PAGE 91 — 12. Root canal condensation
PAGE 99 — 13. Microleakage
PAGE 106 — 14. Endodontic microsurgery
PAGE 114 — 15. Endodontic treatment outcomes
PAGE 121 — 16. Mineral trioxide aggregate
PAGE 128 — 17. Cone-beam computed tomography
PAGE 135 — 18. Pulp revascularization
PAGE 143 — 19. Dental pulp tissue engineering
PAGE 151 — 20. Dental pulp cells

エンドのための重要20キーワード

1 *Pulpitis*

歯髄炎

　歯髄は、細菌感染を生じていなければ、保存できる可能性も高く、そのため、歯髄が保存可能かどうか鑑別診断できることが重要である。不可逆性歯髄炎を生じる前に、歯髄を保護し、歯髄保存療法を行うことは、質の高い歯内療法へとつながる。歯髄炎に関しては、歯髄の細菌感染など、多様な論文が散見される。

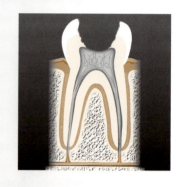

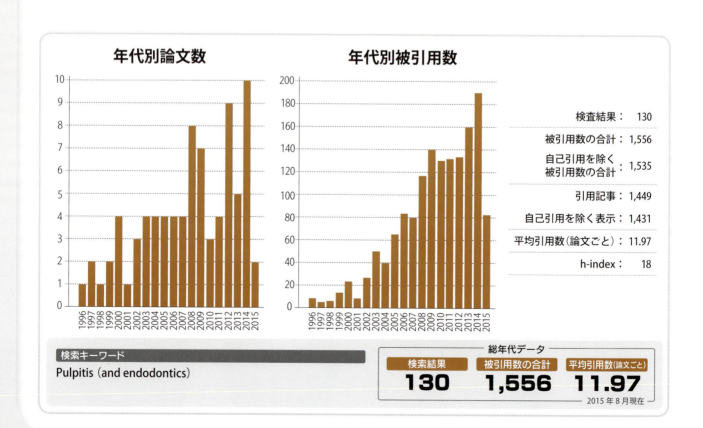

検索キーワード: Pulpitis (and endodontics)

検査結果: 130
被引用数の合計: 1,556
自己引用を除く被引用数の合計: 1,535
引用記事: 1,449
自己引用を除く表示: 1,431
平均引用数(論文ごと): 11.97
h-index: 18

総年代データ
検索結果: 130
被引用数の合計: 1,556
平均引用数(論文ごと): 11.97

2015年8月現在

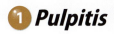

トムソン・ロイターが選んだベスト12論文

	タイトル・和訳	2011年	2012年	2013年	2014年	合計引用数
引用数 1位	Love RM, Jenkinson HF. Invasion of dentinal tubules by oral bacteria. Crit Rev Oral Biol Med 2002；13（2）：171-183. 口腔内細菌による象牙細管の浸潤 本項に和訳あり	10	15	19	23	165
引用数 2位	Nakashima M, Akamine A. The application of tissue engineering to regeneration of pulp and dentin in endodontics. J Endod 2005；31(10)：711-718. 歯内療法における歯髄および象牙質を再生するための組織工学の応用 本項に和訳あり	17	11	16	15	122
引用数 3位	Weiger R, Hitzler S, Hermle G, Löst C. Periapical status, quality of root canal fillings and estimated endodontic treatment needs in an urban German population. Endod Dent Traumatol 1997；13（2）：69-74. ドイツ都市部の住民における根尖周囲の状態、根管充填の質、および推定される根管治療ニーズ量 本項に和訳あり	10	8	7	4	89
引用数 4位	Eriksen HM. Endodontology-epidemiologic considerations. Endod Dent Traumatol 1991；7（5）：189-195. 歯内療法学―疫学的検討 本項に和訳あり	2	1	3	0	60
引用数 5位	Bonsor SJ, Nichol R, Reid TM, Pearson GJ. Microbiological evaluation of photo-activated disinfection in endodontics（an in vivo study）. Br Dent J 2006；200（6）：337-341. 歯内療法における光殺菌に関する微生物学的評価（in vivo での研究） 本項に和訳あり	11	5	4	4	50
引用数 6位	Bender IB. Pulpal pain diagnosis – a review. J Endod 2000；26（3）：175-179. 歯髄痛の診断―総説	1	5	3	6	44

エンドのための重要20キーワード（関連性の高い論文和訳）

トムソン・ロイターが選んだベスト12論文

	タイトル・和訳	2011年	2012年	2013年	2014年	合計引用数
引用数 7位	Iohara K, Imabayashi K, Ishizaka R, Watanabe A, Nabekura J, Ito M, Matsushita K, Nakamura H, Nakashima M. Complete pulp regeneration after pulpectomy by transplantation of CD105+ stem cells with stromal cell-derived factor-1. Tissue Eng Part A 2011；17(15-16)：1911-1920. SDF-1（stromal cell-derived factor-1）を有するCD105陽性幹細胞の移植による抜髄後の完全な歯髄再生	0	6	12	16	39
引用数 8位	Baad-Hansen L. Atypical odontalgia-pathophysiology and clinical management. J Oral Rehabil 2008；35(1)：1-11. 非定型歯痛－病態生理学と臨床管理	2	1	7	6	33
引用数 9位	Hashimura T, Sato M, Hoshino E. Detection of *Slackia exigua*, *Mogibacterium timidum* and *Eubacterium saphenum* from pulpal and periradicular samples using the Polymerase Chain Reaction (PCR) method. Int Endod J 2001；34(6)：463-470. ポリメラーゼ連鎖反応（PCR）法を用いた歯髄および根尖部試料からの*Slackia exigua*菌、*Mogibacterium timidum*菌、および*Eubacterium saphenum*菌の検出	2	3	0	0	26
引用数 10位	Abbott PV, Hume WR, Pearman JW. Antibiotics and endodontics. Aust Dent J 1990；35(1)：50-60. 抗生剤と歯内療法	1	2	1	0	26
引用数 11位	Yingling NM, Byrne BE, Hartwell GR. Antibiotic use by members of the American Association of Endodontists in the year 2000：report of a national survey. J Endod 2002；28(5)：396-404. 西暦2000年における米国歯内療法学会（AAE）会員の抗生剤使用：全国調査報告	1	2	3	3	25
引用数 12位	Gatewood RS, Himel VT, Dorn SO. Treatment of the endodontic emergency：a decade later. J Endod 1990；16(6)：284-291. 歯内療法救急外来における処置：それから10年後について	0	0	1	0	22

Invasion of dentinal tubules by oral bacteria

口腔内細菌による象牙細管の浸潤

Love RM, Jenkinson HF.

　象牙細管の細菌侵入は、エナメル質やセメント質被覆の健全性が侵害され、象牙質が露出したときに、通常、起こる。細菌産生物質は象牙細管を通り歯髄へと拡散し、そして象牙質/歯髄複合体における炎症性変化を惹起する。これらの炎症性変化は、細菌侵襲を排除し、感染ルートを遮断するかもしれない。もし細菌侵入が抑制できなければ、細菌浸潤は、歯髄炎、歯髄壊死、根管系の感染、および根尖病変をもたらすことになる。数百の細菌種が口腔内に存在することが知られている一方で、比較的少なく限られた細菌群が、象牙細管に浸潤し、その後の根管空隙の感染に関与する。う蝕象牙質および健全象牙質の両方において、グラム陽性細菌が細管に存在する微生物のなかで優位である。ユウバクテリウム属、プロピオニバクテリウム属、ビフィドバクテリウム属、ペプトストレプトコッカス‐ミクロス、そしてベイロネラ属といった、比較的多数の偏性嫌気性菌が存在することから、これらの細菌の成長に好ましい環境であることが示唆される。ポルフィロモナス属をはじめとするグラム陰性偏性嫌気性桿菌はそれほど多く回収できなかった。レンサ球菌は、象牙質に侵入する細菌のなかでもっともよく同定される細菌のひとつである。細菌接着および細管内成長を刺激するコラーゲンIなどの象牙細管成分をレンサ球菌が認識していることを、近年の科学的根拠は示唆している。浸潤したレンサ球菌と他の口腔内細菌との特異的な相互作用は、その結果、選択的な細菌分類による象牙質侵入を容易にしている。細菌の象牙細管浸潤にかかわる仕組みを理解することは、歯内療法の実践に役立つ口腔ケア製品や、歯科材料に反映される抑制化合物のような新しい制御法の開発の機会を得られることになるだろう。

（Crit Rev Oral Biol Med 2002；13（2）：171-183.）

Bacterial invasion of dentinal tubules commonly occurs when dentin is exposed following a breach in the integrity of the overlying enamel or cementum. Bacterial products diffuse through the dentinal tubule toward the pulp and evoke inflammatory changes in the pulpo-dentin complex. These may eliminate the bacterial insult and block the route of infection. Unchecked, invasion results in pulpitis and pulp necrosis, infection of the root canal system, and periapical disease. While several hundred bacterial species are known to inhabit the oral cavity, a relatively small and select group of bacteria is involved in the invasion of dentinal tubules and subsequent infection of the root canal space. Gram-positive organisms dominate the tubule microflora in both carious and non-carious dentin. The relatively high numbers of obligate anaerobes present-such as Eubacterium spp., Propionibacterium spp., Bifidobacterium spp., Peptostreptococcus micros, and Veillonella spp.-suggest that the environment favors growth of these bacteria. Gram-negative obligate anaerobic rods, e.g., Porphyromonas spp., are less frequently recovered. Streptococci are among the most commonly identified bacteria that invade dentin. Recent evidence suggests that streptococci may recognize components present within dentinal tubules, such as collagen type I, which stimulate bacterial adhesion and intra-tubular growth. Specific interactions of other oral bacteria with invading streptococci may then facilitate the invasion of dentin by select bacterial groupings. An understanding the mechanisms involved in dentinal tubule invasion by bacteria should allow for the development of new control strategies, such as inhibitory compounds incorporated into oral health care products or dental materials, which would assist in the practice of endodontics.

The application of tissue engineering to regeneration of pulp and dentin in endodontics.

歯内療法における歯髄および象牙質を再生するための組織工学の応用

Nakashima M, Akamine A.

　う蝕、歯髄炎、そして根尖性歯周炎は、医療費そして医療費に付随した経済生産性の損失を増やす。それらは最終的に早期の歯の喪失を生じ、それゆえ、生活の質の低下につながる。歯髄幹細胞/歯髄前駆細胞を用いる生活歯髄療法の進歩は、すべての歯髄を除去することなく象牙質/歯髄複合体の再生を促進できるかもしれない。組織工学は、デザイン科学であり、がんや外傷を含めた疾病により失った部位と入れ替わる新しい組織を製作することである。組織工学の重要な要素は3つあり、形態発生シグナル、モルフォゲンに反応する幹細胞、そして細胞外マトリックスの足場(スキャホールド)である。骨、心臓、肝臓、そして腎臓のような多くの組織や器官において、自然な生物学的再生を加速もしくは誘導するために、前臨床試験における細胞療法や遺伝子治療が、組織障害部位へ足場に移植した幹細胞/前駆細胞とともに成長因子、サイトカイン、およびモルフォゲンを供給するための手段として発展してきた。歯髄組織は、骨形成タンパク質(BMP)に反応して象牙芽細胞に分化する潜在能を有する幹細胞/前駆細胞を含んでいる。象牙質を再生するためには2つの方法がある。1つ目は、*in vivo*における治療法であり、BMPタンパクもしくはBMP遺伝子を露髄した歯髄や生活断髄を行った歯髄に直接適用する。2つ目は、*ex vivo*における治療法であり、歯髄組織からの幹細胞/前駆細胞の単離、遺伝子組み換えBMPやBMP遺伝子を用いた象牙芽細胞への分化、そして、象牙質再生のための最終的な自家移植からなる。本総説はこの領域における近年の進歩について焦点を当て、そして歯内療法における臨床的汎用性への障害と挑戦について考察する。

（J Endod 2005；31(10)：711-718.）

Caries, pulpitis, and apical periodontitis increase health care costs and attendant loss of economic productivity. They ultimately result in premature tooth loss and therefore diminishing the quality of life. Advances in vital pulp therapy with pulp stem/progenitor cells might give impetus to regenerate dentin-pulp complex without the removal of the whole pulp. Tissue engineering is the science of design and manufacture of new tissues to replace lost parts because of diseases including cancer and trauma. The three key ingredients for tissue engineering are signals for morphogenesis, stem cells for responding to morphogens and the scaffold of extracellular matrix. In preclinical studies cell therapy and gene therapy have been developed for many tissues and organs such as bone, heart, liver, and kidney as a means of delivering growth factors, cytokines, or morphogens with stem/progenitor cells in a scaffold to the sites of tissue injury to accelerate and/or induce a natural biological regeneration. The pulp tissue contains stem/progenitor cells that potentially differentiate into odontoblasts in response to bone morphogenetic proteins (BMPs). There are two strategies to regenerate dentin. First, is *in vivo* therapy, where BMP proteins or BMP genes are directly applied to the exposed or amputated pulp. Second is *ex vivo* therapy and consists of isolation of stem/progenitor cells from pulp tissue, differentiation into odontoblasts with recombinant BMPs or BMP genes and finally transplanted autogenously to regenerate dentin. This review is focused on the recent progress in this area and discusses the barriers and challenges for clinical utility in endodontics.

Periapical status, quality of root canal fillings and estimated endodontic treatment needs in an urban German population.

ドイツ都市部の住民における根尖周囲の状態、根管充填の質、および推定される根管治療ニーズ量

Weiger R, Hitzler S, Hermle G, Löst C.

　本研究の目的は、根尖歯周組織の状態、根管充填の質を特定し、そしてドイツ国民における根管治療の必要性を推定することである。臨床データ、エックス線データ、および用いられた術式が、1993年にドイツ・シュトゥットガルトの口腔外科を訪れた患者323名に対して評価された。182名が、少なくとも1歯は根管充填、壊死歯髄、もしくは不可逆性歯髄炎を呈していた。調査した7,897歯のうち、215歯（2.7％）は根管治療の既往があり（カテゴリーA）、122歯（1.5％）は根管治療歴がなく歯髄診に反応しない（カテゴリーB）、そして3歯（0.7％）は不可逆性炎症歯髄組織であると診断された（カテゴリーC）。根尖病変と思われるエックス線像をともなう歯の罹患率は、根管充填歯群において61％、無髄歯でかつ根管治療歴のない群で88％であった。技術標準（テクニカルスタンダード）の評価基準として根管充填の到達度と緊密度を用いたところ、歯根切除術を除く根管治療の既往がある歯の14％だけが、適切と評価された。根管治療が最低限必要とされる症例は、根尖病変の臨床症状をともなう根管充填歯（カテゴリーA）および根尖性歯周炎の臨床症状をともなうカテゴリーBとCを含めた全調査歯において2.3％であった。根尖病変をともなうほとんどの無症状な根管治療歯において根管充填の質が乏しいことを考慮すると、本当に根管治療が必要な症例はもっと多いことが示唆される。これらの歯を再治療した場合、歯内療法が必要なのは3.7％と算出された。

（Endod Dent Traumatol 1997；13（2）：69-74.）

The objective of this study was to determine the periapical status and the quality of root canal fillings and to estimate the endodontic treatment needs in a German population. Clinical and radiographic data and the operative procedures performed were evaluated on 323 patients coming to a dental surgery in Stuttgart, Germany, in 1993. In 182 individuals at least one tooth exhibited a root canal filling, a necrotic pulp or an irreversible pulpitis. Out of the 7,897 teeth examined, 215 (2.7%) had a root canal treatment (category A), 122 being non-endodontically treated (1.5%) did not respond to the sensitivity test (category B) and 53 (0.7%) were diagnosed as having irreversible inflamed pulp tissue (category C). The prevalence of teeth associated with radiographic signs of periapical pathosis was 61% in the group of root canal filled teeth and 88% in the group of pulpless and non-endodontically treated teeth. Using the level and the density of the root canal filling as criteria for evaluating the technical standard, only 14% of the endodontic treatments of non-apicectomized teeth were qualified as adequate. The minimal endodontic treatment need is 2.3% related to all examined teeth when the root canal filled teeth with clinical symptoms of periapical periodontitis (category A) and those of categories B and C are included. The real endodontic treatment need is suggested to be larger when considering that the technical quality of the obturation is poor in most symptomless endodontically treated teeth associated with a periapical lesion. In the case of retreatment of these teeth, the endodontic treatment need would then be calculated at 3.7%.

Endodontology-epidemiologic considerations.

歯内療法学－疫学的検討

Eriksen HM.

　歯内療法疫学調査からの限られた情報ではあるが、加齢にともない根尖病変の罹患率が増加することが示されている。そのうえ根尖病変は、歯内療法処置歯に主にみられるようである。この所見はとくに懸念されるべきで、なぜなら、歯内療法専門医の歯内療法と一般開業医の歯内療法の質と成功率に矛盾があるからである。歯髄炎と急性根尖性歯周炎は、応急処置を求める主たる理由であり、多くの人が罹患している。象牙質/歯髄を含んで起きることの多い歯の外傷は、同様に流行っており、子どもや若者の30％が罹患している。歯内療法に関して見受けられるほとんどの情報が、歯内療法専門医によって巧みに行われた臨床研究から得られたものである。疫学的データは、歯内療法医の成功率を改善するため、病態の原因や適切な治療手技に関した知識の源泉の補完に必要なものである。

（Endod Dent Traumatol 1991；7（5）：189-195.）

The limited information available from endodontic epidemiologic research indicates an increase in prevalence of apical periodontitis with increasing age. Furthermore, apical periodontitis seems mainly to be present in connection with already endodontically treated teeth. This finding should be of particular concern since there is a discrepancy between the quality and results of endodontic therapy performed in general practice compared with the results obtained in specialty clinics. Pulpitis and acute apical periodontitis are main reasons for seeking emergency treatment and affect many people. Dental trauma frequently involving the dentin/pulp organ are likewise prevalent, affecting 30% of children and adolescents. Most information available regarding endodontic treatment is derived from well-controlled clinical studies performed by specialists. Epidemiologic data should be considered a necessary complement to this source of knowledge regarding etiologic factors and proper treatment procedures in order to improve the results of endodontic practice.

Microbiological evaluation of photo-activated disinfection in endodontics (an *in vivo* study).

歯内療法における光殺菌に関する微生物学的評価（*in vivo* での研究）

Bonsor SJ, Nichol R, Reid TM, Pearson GJ.

目的：*in vivo* において通常の根管内感染除去の補助に用いた光殺菌（PAD）の有する微生物学的効果の解明を目的とした。

デザイン：無作為治験が一般歯科開業医で実施された。

対象と方法：歯内療法を必要とする不可逆性歯髄炎あるいは根尖性歯周炎の症状を呈する患者を無作為に抽出した。根管アクセス時、通常の歯内療法後、最後に形成終了後の根管に PAD プロセス（光増感剤と光照射）を施した際に、根管の微生物試料をそれぞれ採取した。それぞれの根管の3つの試料はすべて、試料採取後30分以内にプレートに播種された後、5日間嫌気培養された。細菌量を測定するため、サンプルごとの生菌増殖が記録された。

結果：32根管中30根管の結果を本研究結果に含めた。残り2根管の培養試料は、生存を維持可能な目標時間内に実験室に運ばれなかった。残りの30根管中10根管は培養陰性であった。これらの培養陰性の根管は、培養陰性根管以外の根管に感染がある複根歯の1根管か、または複合抗生剤ペーストの前処置が充血性歯髄炎に行われた複根歯の1根管であった。残った16個は通常の歯内療法後の培養において陰性であった。歯内療法後に感染が除去できなかった4根管中3根管で、PAD プロセス後に培養陰性となった。光送達システムを再点検したところ、培養中に細菌が依然として確認された1根管では、ファイバー破損のため、有効光出力が90％減弱していたことが明らかになった。

結論：歯内療法において PAD システムは従来的な根管洗浄剤使用後に残存した細菌を破壊する手段を提供する。

（Endod Dent Traumatol 1991；7（5）：189-195.）

OBJECTIVE: To determine the microbiological effect of photoactivated disinfection (PAD) as an adjunct to normal root canal disinfection *in vivo*.
DESIGN: A randomised trial carried out in general dental practice.
SUBJECTS AND METHODS: Patients presenting with symptoms of irreversible pulpitis or periradicular periodontitis requiring endodontic therapy were selected at random. A microbiological sample of the canal was taken on accessing the canal, after conventional endodontic therapy, and finally after the PAD process (photosensitiser and light) had been carried out on the prepared canal. All three samples from each canal were plated within 30 minutes of sampling and cultured anaerobically for five days. Growth of viable bacteria was recorded for each sample to determine bacterial load.
RESULTS: Thirty of the 32 canals were included in the results. Cultures from the remaining two did not reach the laboratory within the target time during which viability was sustained. Of the remaining 30, 10 canals were negative to culture. These were either one of the canals in multi rooted teeth where the others were infected or where a pre-treatment with a poly-antibiotic paste had been applied to hyperaemic vital tissue. Sixteen of the remainder were negative to culture after conventional endodontic therapy. Three of the four which had remained infected cultured negative after the PAD process. In the one canal where culturable bacteria were still present, a review of the light delivery system showed a fracture in the fibre reducing the effective light output by 90%.
CONCLUSIONS: The PAD system offers a means of destroying bacteria remaining after using conventional irrigants in endodontic therapy.

エンドのための重要20キーワード

2 *Periapical lesion*
根尖病変

根尖病変は、通常の歯科治療において頻繁に遭遇する疾患のひとつである。根尖病変の本態は、根管経由で侵入してきた細菌や細菌関連物質を、根尖という局所で防御するための生体反応である。この根尖病変の処置を不確実なものとする要因としては、複雑で多様な細菌の感染や、この細菌感染の排除を阻む解剖学形態の複雑性などが挙げられる。本稿では、このような細菌感染について検索した論文を主として紹介する。

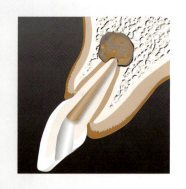

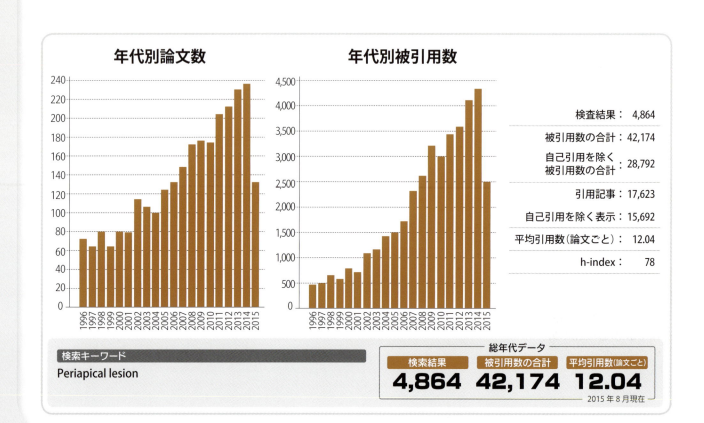

検査結果	4,864
被引用数の合計	42,174
自己引用を除く被引用数の合計	28,792
引用記事	17,623
自己引用を除く表示	15,692
平均引用数（論文ごと）	12.04
h-index	78

検索キーワード: Periapical lesion

総年代データ — 検索結果 4,864／被引用数の合計 42,174／平均引用数（論文ごと）12.04
2015年8月現在

2 Periapical lesion

トムソン・ロイターが選んだベスト12論文

	タイトル・和訳	2011年	2012年	2013年	2014年	合計引用数
引用数 1位	Sundqvist G, Figdor D, Persson S, Sjögren U. Microbiologic analysis of teeth with failed endodontic treatment and the outcome of conservative re-treatment. Oral Surg Oral Med Oral Pathol Oral Radiol Endod 1998；85（1）：86-93. 歯内療法を失敗した歯の細菌学的解析と再保存治療の治療成績 **チャプター15に和訳あり**	31	38	39	36	547
引用数 2位	Sjogren U, Hagglund B, Sundqvist G, Wing K. Factors affecting the long-term results of endodontic treatment. J Endod 1990；16(10)：498-504. 根管治療の長期予後成績に影響する因子 **チャプター15に和訳あり**	33	37	32	35	543
引用数 3位	Byström A, Sundqvist G. Bacteriologic evaluation of the efficacy of mechanical root canal instrumentation in endodontic therapy. Scand J Dent Res 1981；89（4）：321-328. 歯内治療における機械的根管形成の有効性の細菌学的評価 **本項に和訳あり**	23	24	15	14	345
引用数 4位	Nair PN, Sjögren U, Krey G, Kahnberg KE, Sundqvist G. Intraradicular bacteria and fungi in root-filled, asymptomatic human teeth with therapy-resistant periapical lesions：a long-term light and electron microscopic follow-up study. J Endod 1990；16(12)：580-588. 治療耐性を有した根尖病巣の認められるヒト無症状根管充填歯における根管内細菌および真菌：長期にわたる光学および電子顕微鏡による追跡研究	12	12	10	15	277
引用数 5位	Sjögren U, Figdor D, Spångberg L, Sundqvist G. The antimicrobial effect of calcium hydroxide as a short-term intracanal dressing. Int Endod J 1991；24（3）：119-125. 短期間根管貼薬したときの水酸化カルシウムの抗菌効果 **チャプター11に和訳あり**	17	14	15	12	269
引用数 6位	Nair PN, Henry S, Cano V, Vera J. Microbial status of apical root canal system of human mandibular first molars with primary apical periodontitis after "one-visit" endodontic treatment. Oral Surg Oral Med Oral Pathol Oral Radiol Endod 2005；99（2）：231-252. 1回治療法を用いた歯内療法後の初発根尖病変を有するヒト下顎第一大臼歯根尖部根管系の細菌学的状態 **チャプター 8 に和訳あり**	31	27	27	27	256

トムソン・ロイターが選んだベスト**12**論文

	タイトル・和訳	2011年	2012年	2013年	2014年	合計引用数
引用数 **7**位	Nair PN. Pathogenesis of apical periodontitis and the causes of endodontic failures. Crit Rev Oral Biol Med 2004；15（6）：348-381. 根尖性歯周炎の病因および歯内療法の失敗原因 **本項に和訳あり**	30	24	31	33	220
引用数 **8**位	Torabinejad M, Hong CU, Lee SJ, Monsef M, Pitt Ford TR. Investigation of mineral trioxide aggregate for root-end filling in dogs. J Endod 1995；21(12)：603-608. イヌの逆根管充填に用いた mineral trioxide aggregate の研究 **チャプター16に和訳あり**	16	10	5	13	206
引用数 **9**位	Bystrom A, Happonen RP, Sjogren U, Sundqvist G. Healing of periapical lesions of pulpless teeth after endodontic treatment with controlled asepsis. Endod Dent Traumatol 1987；3（2）：58-63. 無菌的環境下で行った歯内療法後の無髄歯の根尖病変治癒 **本項に和訳あり**	13	6	8	5	180
引用数 **10**位	Pinheiro ET, Gomes BP, Ferraz CC, Sousa EL, Teixeira FB, Souza-Filho FJ. Microorganisms from canals of root-filled teeth with periapical lesions. Int Endod J 2003；36（1）：1-11. 根尖病巣を有する根管充填歯根管の微生物 **本項に和訳あり**	16	17	17	14	179
引用数 **11**位	Siqueira JF Jr. Aetiology of root canal treatment failure: why well-treated teeth can fail. Int Endod J 2001；34（1）：1-10. 根管治療失敗の原因論：なぜ十分に治療された歯が失敗するのか	21	13	14	18	167
引用数 **12**位	Kimberly CL, Byers MR. Inflammation of rat molar pulp and periodontium causes increased calcitonin gene-related peptide and axonal sprouting. Anat Rec 1988；222（3）：289-300. ラット臼歯歯髄の炎症や歯周組織の炎症はカルシトニン関連遺伝子の増加と軸索発芽を生じる	2	3	3	2	152

Periapical lesion

Bacteriologic evaluation of the efficacy of mechanical root canal instrumentation in endodontic therapy.

歯内治療における機械的根管形成の有効性の細菌学的評価

Byström A, Sundqvist G.

根尖病巣をともなう17本の単根歯における細菌の存在が、治療の全期間を通して調査された。根管形成時、根管は生理食塩水を用いて根管洗浄された。抗生剤溶液、あるいは貼薬剤としての抗生剤は用いなかった。細菌は、初回治療時に歯から採取したすべての試料で観察された（平均細菌数 4×10^5 個、範囲 $10^2 \sim 10^7$ 個）、そして嫌気性菌は、観察された菌株のうち、それぞれの試料で１％から10.88％の範囲で観察された。もっともよく単離された細菌株は、*Peptostreptococcus micros*、*Peptostreptococcus anaerobius*、*Fusobacterium nucleatum*、*Bacteroides oralis*、*Bacteroides melaninogenicus subsp intermedius*、そして *Eubacterium alactolyticum* であった。機械的根管形成は相当数の細菌数を減少させた。予約治療開始時に採取した試料では、通常 $10^4 \sim 10^6$ 個の細菌が認められたが、治療終了時には $10^2 \sim 10^3$ 個とさらに減少していた。治療期間中に８歯の根管から細菌が取り除かれた。５回連続の治療にもかかわらず、７根管において細菌は除去されなかった。（しかし、）これら細菌の持続感染に関与するような特別な細菌は認められなかった。５回もの治療にもかかわらず、細菌感染を維持した歯は、初回時の試料に多数の細菌が観察された歯であった。

（Scand J Dent Res 1981；89（4）：321-328.）

The presence of bacteria in 17 single-rooted teeth, with periapical lesions, was studied throughout a whole period of treatment. The root canals were irrigated with physiologic saline solution during instrumentation. No antibacterial solutions or dressings were used. Bacteria were found in all initial specimens from the teeth (median number of bacterial cells 4×10^5, range 10^2-10^7) and the number of strains in the specimens ranged from 1 to 10.88% of the strains were anaerobic. The most commonly isolated species were: *Peptostreptococcus micros*, *Peptostreptococcus anaerobius*, *Fusobacterium nucleatum*, *Bacteroides oralis*, *Bacteroides melaninogenicus subsp intermedius* and *Eubacterium alactolyticum*. Mechanical instrumentation reduced the number of bacteria considerably. Specimens taken at the beginning of each appointment usually contained 10^4-10^6 bacterial cells and at the end 10^2-10^3 fewer. Bacteria were eliminated from the root canals of eight teeth during the treatment. In seven root canals bacteria persisted despite treatment on five successive occasions. There was no evidence that specific microorganisms were implicated in these persistent infections. Teeth where the infection persisted despite being treated five times were those with a high number of bacteria in the initial sample.

Pathogenesis of apical periodontitis and the causes of endodontic failures.

根尖性歯周炎の病因および歯内療法の失敗原因

Nair PN.

　根尖性歯周炎は、歯内に関連した感染の結果で生じ、そして根管系から持続的に放出される細菌や細菌関連物質に対する宿主防御反応として形成される。それは、感染した根部歯髄と歯根膜との界面での微生物因子と宿主防御との動的な接触として考えられ、結果として局所における炎症、硬組織吸収、他の根尖歯周組織の破壊を生じ、最終的に、一般的には根尖病変と呼ばれるが、さまざまな病理組織学的分類のある根尖性歯周炎のいずれかへと成熟する。根尖性歯周炎の治療は、根管系の感染疾患であることから、細菌を根絶させるか、または根管系から放出される微生物学的負荷を十分に減らした後、根管充填によって再感染を防止することからなる。その治療は、かなり高い成功率を誇っている。それにもかかわらず、歯内療法は失敗することもある。その失敗の多くは、治療の質によるものがほとんどで、治療術式、そして感染制御と排除に満足いく治療結果が得られなかったときに起こる。最高水準の術式および綿密かつ緻密な治療が行われたときでさえも、失敗は起こることがある。これは既存の機器、材料、そして術式では根管清掃や充填ができない根管領域があるためで、そのため感染が持続してしまう。非常に稀なケースであるが、治療後に病変治癒を妨げるような根尖歯周組織の持続的な炎症を生じてしまうことも、失敗の要因である。歯内療法における失敗の生物学的な原因に関するデータが、さまざまな雑誌で最近散見されている。本論文は、根尖病変の疾病原因に関する包括的な概要を示し、そして術後に無症状であるが根尖透過像としてエックス線写真で観察される歯内療法症例の失敗原因を示すことを意図している。

（Crit Rev Oral Biol Med 2004；15(6)：348-381.）

Apical periodontitis is a sequel to endodontic infection and manifests itself as the host defense response to microbial challenge emanating from the root canal system. It is viewed as a dynamic encounter between microbial factors and host defenses at the interface between infected radicular pulp and periodontal ligament that results in local inflammation, resorption of hard tissues, destruction of other periapical tissues, and eventual formation of various histopathological categories of apical periodontitis, commonly referred to as periapical lesions. The treatment of apical periodontitis, as a disease of root canal infection, consists of eradicating microbes or substantially reducing the microbial load from the root canal and preventing re-infection by orthograde root filling. The treatment has a remarkably high degree of success. Nevertheless, endodontic treatment can fail. Most failures occur when treatment procedures, mostly of a technical nature, have not reached a satisfactory standard for the control and elimination of infection. Even when the highest standards and the most careful procedures are followed, failures still occur. This is because there are root canal regions that cannot be cleaned and obturated with existing equipments, materials, and techniques, and thus, infection can persist. In very rare cases, there are also factors located within the inflamed periapical tissue that can interfere with post-treatment healing of the lesion. The data on the biological causes of endodontic failures are recent and scattered in various journals. This communication is meant to provide a comprehensive overview of the etio-pathogenesis of apical periodontitis and the causes of failed endodontic treatments that can be visualized in radiographs as asymptomatic post-treatment periapical radiolucencies.

Periapical lesion

Healing of periapical lesions of pulpless teeth after endodontic treatment with controlled asepsis.

無菌的環境下で行った
歯内療法後の無髄歯の根尖病変治癒

Bystrom A, Happonen RP, Sjogren U, Sundqvist G.

　綿密な嫌気性菌検査を使用して、根管充填により歯内療法完了前の感染根管から細菌が排除されたことを明らかにした。治療歯の根尖病変治癒は、2年から5年間にわたり予後評価された。79病変の大部分は、完全に治癒もしくは治癒が期待できるくらい小さな病変の大きさに縮小した。5症例は、病変の大きさがまったく変わらないか、もしくはわずかに減少しただけであった。これらの病変のうち2症例は*Actinomyces*や*Arachnid*といった細菌種の存在が示された。別の1症例においては、根尖歯周組織に象牙質削片を認めた。歯内治療中の綿密な細菌学的モニタリングにもかかわらず治癒できなかった根尖病変は、いくつかの症例によっては、根管外の根尖歯周組織で細菌感染を生じたことによるかもしれない。従来の歯内療法では、これらの部位における細菌へのアクセスは不可能である。

（Endod Dent Traumatol 1987；3（2）：58-63.）

Using a careful anaerobic bacteriological technique, bacteria were shown to be eliminated from infected root canals before the endodontic treatment was finished by root filling. Healing of the periapical lesions of the teeth was followed for 2-5 yr. The majority of the 79 lesions healed completely or decreased in size in such a way that they could be expected to heal. In 5 cases there was no or only an insignificant decrease in the size of the lesions. Two of these lesions were shown to contain bacteria of the species Actinomyces or Arachnid. In another case there were dentin chips in the periapical tissue. Periapical lesions which fail to heal in spite of careful bacteriological monitoring of the endodontic treatment may in some cases be due to an establishment of the bacteria outside the root canal in the periapical tissue. In these sites, the bacteria are inaccessible to conventional endodontic treatment.

Microorganisms from canals of root-filled teeth with periapical lesions.

根尖病巣を有する根管充填歯根管の微生物

Pinheiro ET, Gomes BP, Ferraz CC, Sousa EL, Teixeira FB, Souza-Filho FJ.

目的：本研究の目的は、根管治療を失敗した歯の根管内の微生物相を同定し、さまざな微生物種の臨床的特徴との関連を明らかにすることであった。

方法：根尖病変が持続して認められた根管充填歯60歯が、本研究対象として選択された。非外科的再根管治療において、根管充填材は取り除かれ、そして根管から、サンプル抽出を行った。嫌気性菌種を採取するための先進的な微生物学的技法を用いて、微生物のサンプリング、単離、そして微生物種の同定が実施された。臨床的な特徴と微生物学的な所見の関係が検索された。

結果：微生物は51歯から回収された。ほとんどの症例において、根管ごとに1種あるいは2種の細菌株が認められた。単離された微生物種のうち57.4%が、通性嫌気性菌であり、そして83.3%がグラム陽性菌だった。偏性嫌気性菌は、細菌種の42.6%を占め、そしてもっともよく単離された細菌の種類は、*Peptostreptococcus* で、その細菌種は臨床症状と関連していた（P＜0.01）。統計学的に有意な関係は、(a)痛みあるいは痛みの既往歴と複数菌感染あるいは好気性菌との間（P＜0.05）に、(b)打診痛と細菌 *P. intermedia／P. nigrescens* との間（P＜0.05）に、(c)瘻孔と *Streptococcus spp.*（P＜0.001）あるいは *Actinomyces spp.* との間（P＜0.01）に、そして(d)歯冠部が封鎖されていない歯と *Streptococcus spp.*（P＜0.01）あるいは *Candida spp.* との間（P＜0.01）に認められた。

結論：根管治療失敗後の根管内の微生物相は、主に少数のグラム陽性の細菌種に限られていた。通性嫌気性菌、とくに *E. faecalis* が、もっともよく単離された細菌であったが、複数菌感染および偏性嫌気性菌は、臨床症状のある根管充填歯の根管にしばしば認められた。

(Int Endod J 2003；36(1)：1-11.)

AIM: The objective of the present study was to identify the microbial flora within root canals of teeth with failed root-canal treatment and to determine the association of the various species with clinical features.
METHODOLOGY: Sixty root-filled teeth with persisting periapical lesions were selected for this study. During nonsurgical endodontic retreatment, the root-filling material was removed and the canals were sampled. Microbial sampling, isolation and species determination were performed using advanced microbiological techniques for anaerobic species. The association of microbiological findings with clinical features was investigated.
RESULTS: Microorganisms were recovered from 51 teeth. In most cases, one or two strains per canal were found. Of the microbial species isolated, 57.4% were facultative anaerobic species and 83.3% Gram-positive microorganisms. Enterococcus faecalis was the most frequently recovered bacterial species. Obligate anaerobes accounted for 42.6% of the species and the most frequently isolated genera was Peptostreptococcus, which was associated with clinical symptoms (P<0.01). Significant associations were also observed between; (a) pain or history of pain and polymicrobial infections or anaerobes (P<0.05); (b) tenderness to percussion and Prevotella intermedia/ (P<0.05); (c) sinus and Streptococcus spp. (P<0.001) or Actinomyces spp. (P<0.01); (d) coronally unsealed teeth and Streptococcus spp. or Candida spp. (both with P<0.01).
CONCLUSION: The microbial flora in canals after failure of root-canal treatment were limited to a small number of predominantly Gram-positive microbial species. Facultative anaerobes, especially E. faecalis, were the most commonly isolated microorganisms, however, polymicrobial infections and obligate anaerobes were frequently found in canals of symptomatic root-filled teeth.

エンドのための重要20キーワード

3 Vertical root fracture

垂直性歯根破折

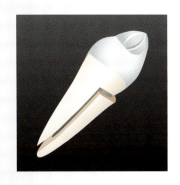

　歯根破折の特徴的な所見として、限局した歯周ポケット、歯肉縁付近の瘻孔、歯根側方の透過像といったことが挙げられる。しかし根尖部に限局した歯根破折などは、歯周ポケットは形成されないこともあり、デンタルエックス線写真だけでは、歯根破折の確定診断をすることは困難な場合も多い。そこで、破折線を、歯科用実体顕微鏡を用いて直接確認することや、歯科用CTを用いて歯根の断面画像を解析することも効果的な診断法と考えられる。本稿では、歯根破折の原因や診断について検索した論文などを紹介する。

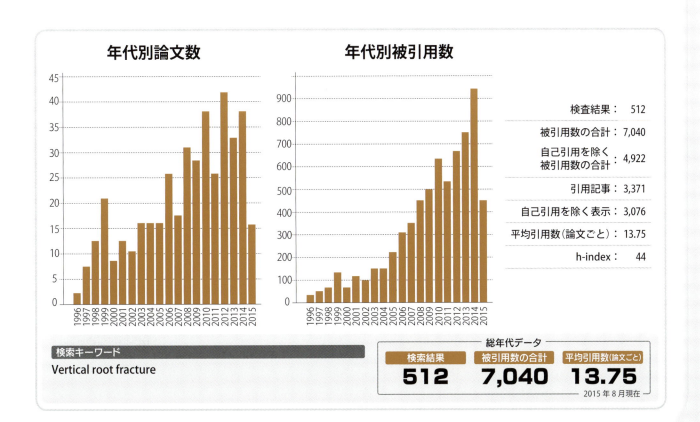

年代別論文数　　年代別被引用数

検査結果：	512
被引用数の合計：	7,040
自己引用を除く被引用数の合計：	4,922
引用記事：	3,371
自己引用を除く表示：	3,076
平均引用数（論文ごと）：	13.75
h-index：	44

検索キーワード
Vertical root fracture

総年代データ
検索結果 512　被引用数の合計 7,040　平均引用数（論文ごと） 13.75
2015年8月現在

エンドのための重要20キーワード（関連性の高い論文和訳）

トムソン・ロイターが選んだベスト**12**論文

	タイトル・和訳	2011年	2012年	2013年	2014年	合計引用数
引用数 1位	Assif D, Gorfil C. Biomechanical considerations in restoring endodontically treated teeth. J Prosthet Dent 1994；71（6）：565-567. 根管治療を受けた歯の修復に関する生体力学的考察 **本項に和訳あり**	11	9	10	10	165
引用数 2位	Teixeira FB, Teixeira EC, Thompson JY, Trope M. Fracture resistance of roots endodontically treated with a new resin filling material. J Am Dent Assoc 2004；135（5）：646-652. 新しいレジン系根管充填材で歯内処置された根管の破折抵抗性 **本項に和訳あり**	9	14	10	9	163
引用数 3位	Meister F Jr, Lommel TJ, Gerstein H. Diagnosis and possible causes of vertical root fractures. Oral Surg Oral Med Oral Pathol 1980；49（3）：243-253. 垂直性歯根破折の診断と原因 **本項に和訳あり**	3	8	6	4	122
引用数 4位	Tamse A, Fuss Z, Lustig J, Kaplavi J. An evaluation of endodontically treated vertically fractured teeth. J Endod 1999；25（7）：506-508. 垂直性歯根破折を生じた歯内治療歯の評価 **本項に和訳あり**	10	12	9	9	96
引用数 5位	Hassan B, Metska ME, Ozok AR, van der Stelt P, Wesselink PR. Detection of vertical root fractures in endodontically treated teeth by a cone beam computed tomography scan. J Endod 2009；35（5）：719-722. 歯内治療歯のコーンビームCTスキャンによる垂直性歯根破折の探索	14	17	17	21	90
引用数 6位	Pitts DL, Natkin E. Diagnosis and treatment of vertical root fractures. J Endod 1983；9（8）：338-346. 垂直性歯根破折の診断および治療	7	2	3	5	86
引用数 7位	Testori T, Badino M, Castagnola M. Vertical root fractures in endodontically treated teeth：a clinical survey of 36 cases. J Endod 1993；19（2）：87-91. 歯内治療歯における垂直性歯根破折：36症例の臨床調査 **本項に和訳あり**	3	5	6	5	81

3 Vertical root fracture

トムソン・ロイターが選んだベスト12論文

	タイトル・和訳	2011年	2012年	2013年	2014年	合計引用数
引用数 8位	Tamse A. Iatrogenic vertical root fractures in endodontically treated teeth. Endod Dent Traumatol 1988；4（5）：190-196. 歯内治療歯における医原性垂直性歯根破折	3	4	4	3	77
引用数 9位	Lertchirakarn V, Palamara JE, Messer HH. Patterns of vertical root fracture：factors affecting stress distribution in the root canal. J Endod 2003；29（8）：523-528. 垂直性歯根破折のパターン：根管の応力分布に影響する因子	5	6	7	13	76
引用数 10位	Tan PL, Aquilino SA, Gratton DG, Stanford CM, Tan SC, Johnson WT, Dawson D. In vitro fracture resistance of endodontically treated central incisors with varying ferrule heights and configurations. J Prosthet Dent 2005；93（4）：331-336. 種々のフェルールの高さと設定条件をもつ歯内治療された中切歯の in vitro における破折抵抗性	3	7	7	15	74
引用数 11位	Morfis AS. Vertical root fractures. Oral Surg Oral Med Oral Pathol 1990；69（5）：631-635. 垂直性歯根破折	2	4	6	4	70
引用数 12位	Holcomb JQ, Pitts DL, Nicholls JI. Further investigation of spreader loads required to cause vertical root fracture during lateral condensation. J Endod 1987；13（6）：277-284. 側方加圧充填時に垂直性歯根破折をきたすことに要するスプレッダー荷重のさらなる研究	4	4	2	4	65

Biomechanical considerations in restoring endodontically treated teeth.

根管治療を受けた歯の修復に関する生体力学的考察

Assif D, Gorfil C.

　歯科診療における種々のコンセプトが、歯内療法後の歯の修復のように、適切な考証なしに確立してしまっている。いくらかの研究者や歯科医師は、歯根を強化するために行うポスト修復を強く推奨している。他の研究では、ポストは歯根を実質的に弱くするので、ポスト修復を避けるべきであると述べている。さらなる取り組みでは、ポストは咬合時の破折抵抗性を改善せず、修復を維持できないと示唆している。そこで本稿では、生体力学的な問題を分析し、推奨される臨床的対応を示す。

（J Prosthet Dent 1994；71（6）：565-567.）

Various concepts for dental treatment have been established without appropriate documentation, such as restoration of endodontically treated teeth. Some researchers and dentists strongly recommend including a post with the restoration to strengthen the root. Other studies have indicated that posts may substantially weaken the roots and should be avoided. An additional approach suggested that the post did not improve the resistance to fracture during occlusion and did not support the restoration. Biomechanical problems are analyzed, and a recommended clinical approach is presented.

Vertical root fracture

Fracture resistance of roots endodontically treated with a new resin filling material.

新しいレジン系根管充填材で歯内処置された根管の破折抵抗性

Teixeira FB, Teixeira EC, Thompson JY, Trope M.

緒言：著者らは、ガッタパーチャもしくは新しいレジン系根管充填材を用いて充填された歯内療法処置歯の破折抵抗性を評価した。

方法：著者らは、80本の単根管抜去歯を用い、以下の5群に無作為に分類した：ガッタパーチャを用いて側方加圧充填もしくは垂直加圧充填した群（グループ1とグループ2）。新しいレジン系根管充填材を用いて側方加圧充填もしくは垂直加圧充填した群（グループ3とグループ4）。根管充填を行わないコントロール群（グループ5）。標本は、湿度100％で2週間保管し、ポリエステルレジンに固定後、破壊荷重試験に供された。

結果：著者らは、実験群間における統計学的有意差（$P < 0.05$）を見出した。新根管充填材使用群は未充填のコントロール群と比べて破壊荷重の平均値が高く、そしてガッタパーチャ使用群はコントロール群と比べて低かった。しかし、(上記の結果に) 有意差は認められなかった。使用した根管充填の術式にかかわらず、新根管充填材使用群はガッタパーチャ使用群よりも有意に破折荷重の平均値が高かった。

結論：新レジン系根管充填材を使用して根管充填すると、標準的なガッタパーチャ充填法と比較して、歯内治療を行った単根抜去歯の破折抵抗性は、*in vitro* において増加した。

臨床的な意味：本研究結果が、新レジン系根管充填材を用いると歯の破折抵抗性が増加することを提示できたように、その新レジン系根管充填材の破折抵抗性以外の特性が、ガッタパーチャ根管充填材の特性と比較してさらに良好なものであるならば、ガッタパーチャに取って代わるべき材料として考慮すべきである。

（J Am Dent Assoc 2004；135（5）：646-652.）

BACKGROUND: The authors evaluated the fracture resistance of endodontically treated teeth filled with either gutta-percha or a new resin-based obturation material.
METHODS: The authors prepared and randomly divided 80 single-canal extracted teeth into five groups: lateral and vertical condensation with gutta-percha, lateral and vertical condensation with the new resin-based obturation material, and a control group with no filling material. The specimens were stored in 100 percent humidity for two weeks, mounted in polyester resin and loaded to failure.
RESULTS: The authors found statistically significant differences among the experimental groups (P<.05). The groups with the new material displayed higher mean fracture loads and the gutta-percha groups lower mean fracture load values than the control unfilled group. However, the differences were not significant. The groups with the new material displayed significantly higher mean fracture loads than gutta-percha groups independent of the filling technique used.
CONCLUSIONS: Filling the canals with the new resin-based obturation material increased the *in vitro* resistance to fracture of endodontically treated single-canal extracted teeth when compared with standard gutta-percha techniques.
CLINICAL IMPLICATIONS: If other properties of the new resin-based obturation material compare favorably with those of gutta-percha for filling the root canal, it should be considered as a replacement for gutta-percha, as the results of this study indicate that it could provide enhanced resistance to tooth fracture.

Diagnosis and possible causes of vertical root fractures.

垂直性歯根破折の診断と原因

Meister F Jr, Lommel TJ, Gerstein H.

　垂直性破折を起こした32症例を、日常臨床で見受けられる垂直性破折の破折原因と診断所見を特定するために検討した。2名を除くすべての患者において、骨欠損が存在し、そして探知可能であった。大部分の患者（65.63％）は軽度の痛みや鈍い不快症状を有していた。75％は歯根膜腔の広範な拡大を示した。本研究は、ガッタパーチャ側方加圧時の過度な力が本研究の破折歯84.38％の原因であったと示唆している。2番目の原因はインレーやポストを窩洞へ無理に押し込むことや叩くことであった。患者の大部分（78.13％）は40歳以上であった。9症例を除くすべて症例において、処置は罹患歯の抜歯であった。

（Oral Surg Oral Med Oral Pathol 1980；49(33)：243-253.）

Thirty-two cases of vertical fractures were studied in an attempt to identify the causes and diagnostic signs normally present. In all of the patients except two, osseous defects were present and could be probed. The majortiy (65.63%) had only mild pain or a dull discomfort. Seventy-five percent showed diffuse widening of the periodontal ligament space. This study suggests that excessive force during lateral condensation of the gutta-percha caused 84.38% of the fractures. A secondary cause was the forcing or tapping of inlays or dowels into place. The majority (78.13%) of the patients were over the age of 40. In all but nine of the cases, treatment consisted of the extraction of the involved teeth,

An evaluation of endodontically treated vertically fractured teeth.

垂直性歯根破折を生じた歯内治療歯の評価

Tamse A, Fuss Z, Lustig J, Kaplavi J.

　本調査では、垂直性歯根破折を生じた歯内治療歯92本を、抜歯前後で臨床的・エックス線写真的に評価した。上顎第二小臼歯（27.2％）と下顎大臼歯近心根（24％）は、もっとも破折を生じた歯であった。これらの破折歯の67.4％において、孤立した歯周ポケットが頬側に存在し、34.8％において、瘻孔は根尖部よりも歯肉縁付近で頻繁に出現した。半数以上の症例で、根の側方のエックス線透過像を認めるか、あるいは根の側方と根尖部の両方にエックス線透過像を認めた。一般開業医は、本調査の破折歯92本のうち1/3のみ、垂直性歯根破折と正確に診断できた。

(J Endod 1999 ; 25(7) : 506-508.)

For this survey, 92 vertically fractured endodontically treated teeth were evaluated clinically and radiographically before and after extraction. The maxillary second premolars (27.2%) and mesial roots of the mandibular molars (24%) were the most fractured teeth. In 67.4% of the teeth, a solitary buccal pocket was present: in 34.8%, a fistula frequently appeared closer to the gingival margin than to the apical area. A lateral radiolucency or a combination of lateral and periapical radiolucency was found in more than half of the cases. The general practitioners correctly diagnosed vertical root fracture in only one-third of the 92 fractured teeth in this survey.

Vertical root fractures in endodontically treated teeth: a clinical survey of 36 cases.

歯内治療歯における垂直性歯根破折：36症例の臨床調査

Testori T, Badino M, Castagnola M.

　過去に発表された文献の32症例から収集したデータに沿って、垂直性歯根破折を起こした36症例について臨床研究を実施した。垂直性歯根破折は45歳から60歳の患者の臼歯でもっとも多く生じていた。歯内療法を受けてから、その後垂直性破折と診断されるまでの平均経過時間はおよそ10年であるとわかった。その所見および症状は、たいてい、歯周囲の付着歯肉に生じた1か所だけの深いポケットや、しばしば腫脹と瘻孔をともなうが、破折歯周囲の軽度の痛みであった。エックス線写真でもっともよく認められる所見は、根尖周囲の暈（かさ、ハロー）状の透過像である。

(J Endod 1993;19(2):87-91.)

A clinical study was done on 36 original cases of vertical root fractures along with the data gathered from 32 cases published previously in the literature. Vertical root fractures most frequently occur in posterior teeth in patients between 45 and 60 yr of age. The average elapsed time between the endodontic treatment and the subsequent diagnosis of vertical fracture was found to be approximately 10 yr. The evidence and symptoms most often found are mild pain in the area of the fractured tooth often accompanied by swelling and fistula, along with a deep pocket in just one area of the attachment surrounding the tooth. The sign most often revealed by X-ray is a radiolucent periradicular band.

エンドのための重要20キーワード

4 Apex locators
根管長測定器

根尖孔の位置を特定するために、電気的に根管長を測定する方法は、東京医科歯科大学の砂田今男により、1958年に報告された。その後、2波長相対値法を用いた機器が開発され、日本国内で広く普及するようになる。電気的根管長測定モジュールに、Ni-Ti製ファイルを用いた根管形成のモジュールを付加した新世代の電気的根管長測定器も登場している。論文としては、ファイルの先端と根尖孔との位置関係を、各種電気的根管長測定器のインピーダンスに関して、測定の正確性を検索した論文が多数発表されている。

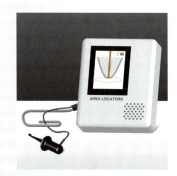

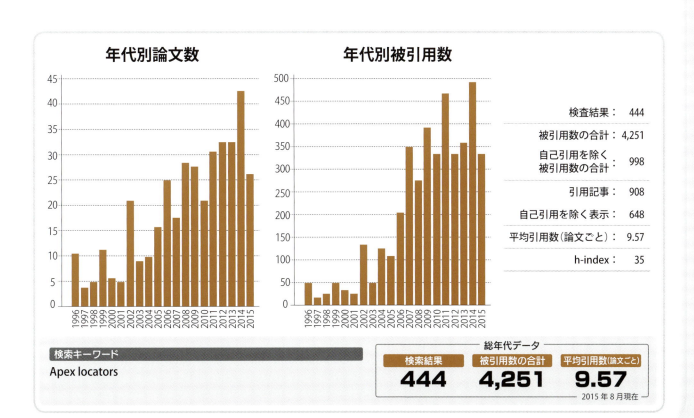

年代別論文数 / **年代別被引用数**

検査結果	444
被引用数の合計	4,251
自己引用を除く被引用数の合計	998
引用記事	908
自己引用を除く表示	648
平均引用数（論文ごと）	9.57
h-index	35

検索キーワード: Apex locators

総年代データ
- 検査結果: 444
- 被引用数の合計: 4,251
- 平均引用数（論文ごと）: 9.57

2015年8月現在

エンドのための重要20キーワード（関連性の高い論文和訳）

トムソン・ロイターが選んだベスト**12**論文

	タイトル・和訳	2011年	2012年	2013年	2014年	合計引用数
引用数 **1**位	Gordon MP, Chandler NP. Electronic apex locators. Int Endod J 2004 ; 37（7）: 425-437. 電気的根管長測定器	17	9	11	10	100
引用数 **2**位	Shabahang S, Goon WW, Gluskin AH. An *in vivo* evaluation of Root ZX electronic apex locator. J Endod 1996 ; 22(11) : 616-618. Root ZX 電気的根管長測定器の *in vivo* における評価	12	6	4	6	100
引用数 **3**位	Kobayashi C, Suda H. New electronic canal measuring device based on the ratio method. J Endod 1994 ; 20（3）: 111-114. 比率法に基づく新しい電気的根管長測定器 **本項に和訳あり**	9	3	2	5	95
引用数 **4**位	Nekoofar MH, Ghandi MM, Hayes SJ, Dummer PM. The fundamental operating principles of electronic root canal length measurement devices. Int Endod J 2006 ; 39（8）: 595-609. 電気的根管長測定器の基本的な動作原理 **本項に和訳あり**	13	6	8	9	69
引用数 **5**位	Plotino G, Grande NM, Brigante L, Lesti B, Somma F. *Ex vivo* accuracy of three electronic apex locators : Root ZX, Elements Diagnostic Unit and Apex Locator and ProPex. Int Endod J 2006 ; 39（5）: 408-414. 3 機種の電気的根管長測定器の *ex vivo* における精度：Root ZX、Elements Diagnostic Unit and Apex Locator、および ProPex **本項に和訳あり**	9	5	2	5	54
引用数 **6**位	Wrbas KT, Ziegler AA, Altenburger MJ, Schirrmeister JF. *In vivo* comparison of working length determination with two electronic apex locators. Int Endod J 2007 ; 40（2）: 133-138. 電気的根管長測定器 2 機種を用いた作業長測定の *in vivo* における比較 **本項に和訳あり**	8	5	5	5	48
引用数 **7**位	Hoer D, Attin T. The accuracy of electronic working length determination. Int Endod J 2004 ; 37（2）: 125-131. 電気的な作業長測定の精度	5	4	3	3	44

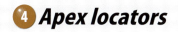

トムソン・ロイターが選んだベスト12論文

	タイトル・和訳	2011年	2012年	2013年	2014年	合計引用数
引用数 8位	Jenkins JA, Walker WA 3 rd, Schindler WG, Flores CM. An *in vitro* evaluation of the accuracy of the Root ZX in the presence of various irrigants. J Endod 2001；27（3）：209-211. 種々の根管洗浄剤の存在下におけるRoot ZXの精度に関する*in vitro*評価 **本項に和訳あり**	2	2	3	2	42
引用数 9位	Williams CB, Joyce AP, Roberts S. A comparison between *in vivo* radiographic working length determination and measurement after extraction. J Endod 2006；32（7）：624-627. *in vivo*におけるエックス線写真を用いた作業長測定と抜歯後の測定との比較	9	4	3	6	36
引用数 10位	Stein TJ, Corcoran JF. Radiographic "working length" revisited. Oral Surg Oral Med Oral Pathol 1992；74（6）：796-800. エックス線写真での"作業長"の再検討	3	2	3	2	36
引用数 11位	Kim E, Lee SJ. Electronic apex locator. Dent Clin North Am 2004；48（1）：35-54. 電気的根管長測定器	4	3	3	2	35
引用数 12位	Kielbassa AM, Muller U, Munz I, Monting JS. Clinical evaluation of the measuring accuracy of ROOT ZX in primary teeth. Oral Surg Oral Med Oral Pathol Oral Radiol Endod 2003；95（1）：94-100. 乳歯におけるROOT ZXの計測精度に関する臨床評価	6	1	2	2	32

New electronic canal measuring device based on the ratio method.

比率法に基づく新しい電気的根管長測定器

Kobayashi C, Suda H.

　ほとんどの根管長測定器のもっとも著しく不都合な点は、根管内に電解液があった場合に、測定器の表示が短すぎる値を示し、ときには測定自体ができなくなってしまうことである。この欠点を克服するために、根管長を電気的に測定するための新しいコンセプトが開発された。その装置は、異なる2つの周波数の電流源を用いて2つの根管インピーダンスを同時に測定する。それから、それぞれのインピーダンスに比例する2電位間の割合を算定する。その指数（商）は、装置のメータに表示され、根管のファイル先端の位置を示すこととなる。その指数は根管の電解液にごくわずかに影響されること、そして根尖孔にファイルの先端が近づくと大幅に減少することが、本研究でわかった。

（J Endod 1994；20（3）：111-114.）

> The most striking disadvantage of most apex locators is that if there are electrolytes in the canal the meter shows a reading which is too short or sometimes the measurement itself becomes impossible. To overcome this drawback, a new concept for electrically measuring the root canal length has been developed. The device simultaneously measures two impedances of the canal using current sources with two different frequencies. Then the ratio between the two electric potentials proportional to each impedance is calculated. The quotient is shown on the device's meter and represents the position of a file tip in the canal. The present study found that the quotient was only negligibly influenced by the electrolyte present in the canal and decreased considerably as the file tip approached the apical foramen.

The fundamental operating principles of electronic root canal length measurement devices.

電気的根管長測定器の基本的な動作原理

Nekoofar MH, Ghandi MM, Hayes SJ, Dummer PM.

　根管治療を根管内に制限すべきであることは一般的に受け入れられている。この目的を達成するためには根管形成の間、根端を正確に測定しなければならず、そして根管形成中は厳密に測定した作業長を維持しなければならない。電気的な方法を含むいくつかの測定法が根端の決定のために用いられている。しかしながら、この根管長測定に用いられる電気的装置の基本的な作動原理および分類は、しばしばはっきりせずに、議論の的となる。すべての電気的根管長測定器の基本前提は、ヒト組織が電子部品を組み合わせることにより模造可能な特徴をいくつか備えていることにある。したがって、この模型の抵抗力やインピーダンスといった電気特性を測定することより、根端を探知できるはずである。根管系は、電流の絶縁体である象牙質やセメント質に囲まれている。しかしながら、それ自体が電流の伝導体である歯根膜と電気的につぐ根管腔の導電物質（組織、組織液）を入れた小さな穴である。こうして、根管内の組織や組織液と一体になった象牙質は、象牙質の厚さや真性抵抗率による値を示す抵抗器を形成し、これらの容積により決まる値、固有抵抗率を生じる。歯内療法用ファイルが根管に挿入され、根尖最狭窄部に近づくと、抵抗物質（象牙質、組織、組織液）の有効長が減少するため、歯内療法用ファイルと根尖孔間の抵抗が減少する。抵抗特性と同様に、歯根の構造は容量特性をもっている。したがって、根端を決定するために他のいろいろな原理を用いた種々の電気的手法が開発されている。一番簡単な装置が抵抗を計測する一方、他の装置は高周波、2帯域周波、もしくは多重周波などを用いてインピーダンス測定を行う。さらに、いくつかのシステムは、根端を決定するために低周波振動を用い、あるいは低周波振動と電圧勾配法の両方を使用している。本総説の目的は、根管長測定をうたう異なるタイプの電気システムの基本的な作動原理を明らかにすることであった。

（Int Endod J 2006；39（8）：595-609.）

It is generally accepted that root canal treatment procedures should be confined within the root canal system. To achieve this objective the canal terminus must be detected accurately during canal preparation and precise control of working length during the process must be maintained. Several techniques have been used for determining the apical canal terminus including electronic methods. However, the fundamental electronic operating principles and classification of the electronic devices used in this method are often unknown and a matter of controversy. The basic assumption with all electronic length measuring devices is that human tissues have certain characteristics that can be modelled by a combination of electrical components. Therefore, by measuring the electrical properties of the model, such as resistance and impedance, it should be possible to detect the canal terminus. The root canal system is surrounded by dentine and cementum that are insulators to electrical current. At the minor apical foramen, however, there is a small hole in which conductive materials within the canal space (tissue, fluid) are electrically connected to the periodontal ligament that is itself a conductor of electric current. Thus, dentine, along with tissue and fluid inside the canal, forms a resistor, the value of which depends on their dimensions, and their inherent resistivity. When an endodontic file penetrates inside the canal and approaches the minor apical foramen, the resistance between the endodontic file and the foramen decreases, because the effective length of the resistive material (dentine, tissue, fluid) decreases. As well as resistive properties, the structure of the tooth root has capacitive characteristics. Therefore, various electronic methods have been developed that use a variety of other principles to detect the canal terminus. Whilst the simplest devices measure resistance, other devices measure impedance using either high frequency, two frequencies or multiple frequencies. In addition, some systems use low frequency oscillation and/or a voltage gradient method to detect the canal terminus. The aim of this review was to clarify the fundamental operating principles of the different types of electronic systems that claim to measure canal length.

Ex vivo accuracy of three electronic apex locators : Root ZX, Elements Diagnostic Unit and Apex Locator and ProPex.

3機種の電気的根管長測定器の *ex vivo* における精度：Root ZX、Elements Diagnostic Unit and Apex Locator および ProPex

Plotino G, Grande NM, Brigante L, Lesti B, Somma F.

目的：3機種の根管長測定器、Root ZX、Elements Diagnostic Unit and Apex Locator、および ProPex の精度を *ex vivo* において比較することを本研究の目的とした。

方法：電気的作業長測定は *ex vivo* モデルを用いた40本の抜去歯で行われた。最初の術者は、開拡後、双眼実体顕微鏡の30倍の拡大視野下で、根尖の示標を根尖最狭窄部とし、それぞれの歯の基準長を測定した。その後、すべての歯を各根管長測定器で測定し、得られた測定結果を対応する基準長と比較した。各根管長測定器で電気的に計測した長さから基準長を差し引いた長さを求めた。基準長を超えた計測値は正（長い）と、基準長より短い計測値では負と記録された。グループ間のノンパラメトリックな相関関係に対して Friedman 検定と Tukey 多重範囲検定を用いた統計学的データ解析を行った。$P<0.05$を統計学的に有意とした。

結果：3種の根管長測定器と実体顕微鏡の計測値間の長さの差を比較すると、基準長から±0.5mm以内であった割合は、Root ZXでは97.37％（84.22％は基準長より0.5mm以内短い）、Elementsでは94.28％（88.57％は基準長より0.5mm以内短い）、そして ProPex では100％（35.9％は基準長より0.5mm以内短い）であった。Root ZX、Elements、そして ProPex のそれぞれで測定した長さと、基準長との差の平均値は、それぞれ−0.157±0.228mm、−0.103±0.359mm、0.307±0.271mm であった。

結論：本研究の結果から、根管長測定器は多くの場合において根尖最狭窄部から±0.5mm以内を根管長として測定することがわかった。ProPex による測定は、多くの場合、実際の根管長より長く測定されていた。

(Int Endod J 2006；39（5）：408-414.)

AIM: To compare *ex vivo* the accuracy of three electronic apex locators (EALs): Root ZX, Elements Diagnostic Unit and Apex Locator and ProPex.
METHODOLOGY: Electronic working length determination was carried out in 40 extracted teeth using an *ex vivo* model. After access preparation, a first operator determined the reference length (AL) for each tooth under a 30× stereomicroscope using the apical constriction as the apical landmark. All teeth were then measured with each EAL and the results obtained were compared with the corresponding AL. The AL was subtracted from the electronically determined distance. The measurements exceeding the AL were recorded as positive (long) and the measurements short of the AL were recorded as negative. Data were analyzed using the Friedman Test and Tukey multiple range test for nonparametric correlation amongst groups. Statistical significance was considered at P<0.05.
RESULTS: Comparing the differences between measurements obtained with the three EALs and those obtained with the stereomicroscope, the percentage of measurements within +/-0.5mm of the AL was 97.37% (84.22% within 0.5mm short of AL) for the Root ZX, 94.28% (88.57% within 0.5mm short of AL) for the Elements and 100% (35.9% within 0.5mm short of AL) for the ProPex. The mean difference between the AL and the lengths measured by the Root ZX, the Elements and the ProPex were, respectively, -0.157+/-0.228, -0.103+/-0.359 and 0.307+/-0.271mm.
CONCLUSIONS: The results of the present study confirm that the EALs determined the canal length within +/-0.5mm from the apical constriction in the majority of cases. The majority of the ProPex readings were long.

In vivo comparison of working length determination with two electronic apex locators.

電気的根管長測定器2機種を用いた作業長測定の *in vivo* における比較

Wrbas KT, Ziegler AA, Altenburger MJ, Schirrmeister JF.

目的：2機種の電気的根管長測定器の精度を、同一歯を用いて *in vivo* における比較を行うことを本研究の目的とした。

方法：抜歯前に、異なる2種の電気的根管長測定器(Root ZX、および Raypex 5 VDW)を用いて20本の単根歯の作業長が測定された。1機種目の電気的根管長測定器の使用時には、測定器の画面が"根尖狭窄部"を示すまでファイルを進めた。その後、ファイルは、取り外しや置き換えの可能な光硬化型コンポジット製の鋳型に固定された。この手順は、同一歯において、2機種目の電気的根管長測定器と最初の実験とは異なるファイルを用いて、繰り返し行われた。その後、それらの歯を抜歯し、そして根尖から4mmまでの根管を露出させた。その後、光学顕微鏡下において、もとの位置に復位させたファイルと根尖部のデジタル写真を撮影した。デジタル画像上にて、各標本の最小半径と根尖孔を記録した後、コンピュータプログラムを用いてこれらの位置からファイルの先端までのそれぞれの長さを測定した。その後、2種の電気的根管長測定器を使用した2つの実験群の値は対応のあるT検定により比較された。

結果：根尖最狭窄部は Root ZX の場合75％が、Raypex 5 の場合80％が±0.5mm の範囲内に位置していた。対応のあるT検定によると、根尖最狭窄部の決定に関してそれぞれの電気的根管長測定器間の統計学的有意差は認められなかった。

結論：作業長の決定に、電気的根管長測定器を用いることは、信頼のおける方法である。2種の電気的根管長測定器間の差に、統計学的有意差は認められなかった。

（Int Endod J 2007；40（2）：133-138.）

AIM: To compare the accuracy of two electronic apex locators (EALs) in the same teeth *in vivo*.
METHODOLOGY: The working lengths in 20 teeth with a single canal were determined with two different EALs (Root ZX; J. Morita Corporation, Tokyo, Japan and Raypex 5 VDW, Munich, Germany) before extraction. When the first EAL was used the files were advanced until the display indicated the "apical constriction". The files were then fixed in removable and replaceable light curing composite patterns. The procedure was repeated in the same tooth with the second EAL and a different file. The teeth were then extracted and the apical 4 mm of the root canals were exposed. After that the apical parts with the repositioned files in the canals were digitally photographed under a light microscope. On the images the minor diameter and the major foramen of each sample were marked and the respective distances of the file tips from these positions were measured with a computer program. Subsequently the values of the two groups of EALs were compared using a paired sample t-test.
RESULTS:The minor foramen was located within the limits of +/-0.5mm in 75% of the cases with the Root ZX and in 80% of the cases with Raypex 5. The paired sample t-test showed no significant difference between the EALs regarding determination of the minor foramen.
CONCLUSION: The use of EALs is a reliable method for determining working length. The differences between the two EALs were not statistically significant.

An *in vitro* evaluation of the accuracy of the Root ZX in the presence of various irrigants.

種々の根管洗浄剤の存在下における Root ZX の精度に関する *in vitro* 評価

Jenkins JA, Walker WA 3rd, Schindler WG, Flores CM.

　本研究の目的は、種々の根管洗浄剤の存在下における Root ZX の精度を *in vitro* において評価することである。本研究の *in vitro* モデルは、Donnelly の記述によるもので、水の代わりに0.9％塩化ナトリウムを入れて作成した凍結ゼラチンよりなっていた。以下の根管洗浄剤；エピネフリン8万分の1添加2％リドカイン、5.25％次亜塩素酸ナトリウム、RC Prep、EDTA 溶液、3％過酸化水素水、および Peridex 洗口液を試験した。計30本の単根抜去歯を用いた。種々の根管洗浄剤下における実験の測定値は、実際の根管長と比較された。電気的根管長測定器 Root ZX は0.31mm の範囲内で根管長を正確に測定すること、そして検索した7種の洗浄剤に応じた根管長測定における差はほとんどないことを本研究データは示していた。これらの結果は、Root ZX は歯内療法開業医において一般的に使用されている多岐にわたる洗浄剤を賄える根管長測定に有用で、多用途かつ正確な機器であるという考えを強く支持するものである。

（J Endod 2001；27（3）：209-211.）

The purpose of this study was to evaluate the accuracy of the Root ZX *in vitro* in the presence of a variety of endodontic irrigants. The *in vitro* model, described by Donnelly, consisted of refrigerated gelatin made with 0.9%sodium chloride instead of water. The following irrigants were tested: 2% lidocaine with 1:100,000 epinephrine, 5.25% sodium hypochlorite, RC Prep, liquid EDTA, 3% hydrogen peroxide, and Peridex. A total of 30 extracted, single-rooted teeth were used. The experimental measurements in the presence of the various irrigants were compared with the actual canal lengths. The present data indicate that the Root ZX electronic apex locator reliably measured canal lengths to within 0.31mm and that there was virtually no difference in the length determination as a function of the seven irrigants used. These results strongly support the concept that the Root ZX is a useful, versatile, and accurate device for the determination of canal lengths over a wide range of irrigants commonly used in the practice of endodontics.

エンドのための重要20キーワード

5 Rotary nickel-titanium instruments

Ni-Ti 製ロータリーファイル

歯内療法において、根管形成はもっとも重要なステップである。これまでに開発されてきた根管形成器具のなかで、もっとも革新的な器具の1つにNi-Ti 製ファイルが挙げられる。このファイルの特徴は、曲がりがしなやかであり、力が除かれると元の形状に戻る超弾性効果を有することである。そのための利点として、湾曲根管においても、根管の形態に忠実に、少ない削除量で、速やかに形成可能なことが挙げられる。本項では、さまざまに試みられてきたNi-Ti 製ファイルの論文を紹介することとする。

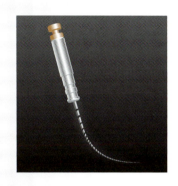

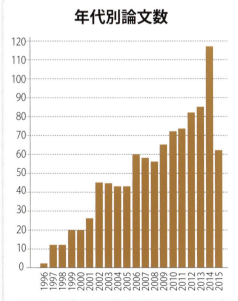

年代別論文数

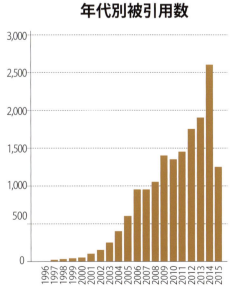

年代別被引用数

検査結果：	1,014
被引用数の合計：	16,627
自己引用を除く被引用数の合計：	6,890
引用記事：	3,221
自己引用を除く表示：	2,459
平均引用数（論文ごと）：	16.40
h-index：	58

検索キーワード
Rotary nickel-titanium instruments

総年代データ

検索結果	被引用数の合計	平均引用数（論文ごと）
1,014	16,627	16.40

2015 年 8 月現在

トムソン・ロイターが選んだベスト12論文

タイトル・和訳	2011年	2012年	2013年	2014年	合計引用数
引用数1位 Pruett JP, Clement DJ, Carnes DL Jr. Cyclic fatigue testing of nickel-titanium endodontic instruments. J Endod 1997；23（2）：77-85. 根管形成用 Ni-Ti 製ファイルの繰り返し疲労試験 チャプター6に和訳あり	23	36	26	27	360
引用数2位 Peters OA. Current challenges and concepts in the preparation of root canal systems：a review. J Endod 2004；30（8）：559-567. 根管系の形成における現在の挑戦とコンセプト：総説論文 チャプター15に和訳あり	28	29	30	41	275
引用数3位 Nair PN, Henry S, Cano V, Vera J. Microbial status of apical root canal system of human mandibular first molars with primary apical periodontitis after "one-visit" endodontic treatment. Oral Surg Oral Med Oral Pathol Oral Radiol Endod 2005；99（2）：231-252. 1回治療法を用いた歯内療法後の初発根尖病変を有するヒト下顎第一大臼歯根尖部根管系の細菌学的状態 チャプター8に和訳あり	31	27	27	27	256
引用数4位 Sattapan B, Nervo GJ, Palamara JE, Messer HH. Defects in rotary nickel-titanium files after clinical use. J Endod 2000；26（3）：161-165. 臨床使用後の Ni-Ti 製ロータリーファイル欠損 チャプター6に和訳あり	20	22	22	37	243
引用数5位 Peters OA, Schönenberger K, Laib A. Effects of four Ni-Ti preparation techniques on root canal geometry assessed by micro computed tomography. Int Endod J 2001；34（3）：221-230. マイクロ CT により評価された4種の Ni-Ti 製ファイルによる根管形成手技の根管形態に対する影響 チャプター7に和訳あり	17	23	21	29	189
引用数6位 Torabinejad M, Khademi AA, Babagoli J, Cho Y, Johnson WB, Bozhilov K, Kim J, Shabahang S. A new solution for the removal of the smear layer. J Endod 2003；29（3）：170-175. スメアー層除去に対する新溶液	16	19	19	9	177

5 Rotary nickel-titanium instruments

トムソン・ロイターが選んだベスト12論文

順位	タイトル・和訳	2011年	2012年	2013年	2014年	合計引用数
引用数 7位	Hülsmann M, Heckendorff M, Lennon A. Chelating agents in root canal treatment : mode of action and indications for their use. Int Endod J 2003 ; 36(12) : 810-830. 根管治療におけるキレート剤：作用機序と使用指針 **チャプター10に和訳あり**	14	16	19	14	143
引用数 8位	Peters OA, Peters CI, Schönenberger K, Barbakow F. ProTaper rotary root canal preparation : effects of canal anatomy on final shape analysed by micro CT. Int Endod J 2003 ; 36(2) : 86-92. **ProTaper**ロータリーファイルによる根管形成：最終形成が根管解剖に及ぼす影響についてのマイクロCTによる評価 **本項に和訳あり**	15	21	8	16	142
引用数 9位	Haïkel Y, Serfaty R, Bateman G, Senger B, Allemann C. Dynamic and cyclic fatigue of engine-driven rotary nickel-titanium endodontic instruments. J Endod 1999 ; 25(6) : 434-440. 歯内療法用Ni-Ti製ロータリーエンジンファイルの動的疲労と繰り返し疲労 **本項に和訳あり**	11	8	12	9	142
引用数 10位	Parashos P, Messer HH. Rotary NiTi instrument fracture and its consequences. J Endod 2006 ; 32(11) : 1031-1043. Ni-Ti製ロータリーファイルの破折とその原因 **本項に和訳あり**	19	14	20	21	133
引用数 11位	Peters OA, Laib A, Göhring TN, Barbakow F. Changes in root canal geometry after preparation assessed by high-resolution computed tomography. J Endod 2001 ; 27(1) : 1-6. 高解像度CTにより評価された根管形成後の根管形態の変化 **チャプター7に和訳あり**	13	12	13	10	125
引用数 12位	Thompson SA, Dummer PM. Shaping ability of ProFile.04 Taper Series 29 rotary nickel-titanium instruments in simulated root canals. Part 1. Int Endod J 1997 ; 30(1) : 1-7. **ProFile.04 Series29 Ni-Ti**製ロータリーファイルの模擬根管における根管形成能。パート1 **本項に和訳あり**	7	1	4	2	106

ProTaper rotary root canal preparation: effects of canal anatomy on final shape analysed by micro CT.

ProTaperロータリーファイルによる根管形成：最終形成が根管解剖に及ぼす影響についてのマイクロCTによる評価

Peters OA, Peters CI, Schönenberger K, Barbakow F.

目的：術前形状のさまざまな根管を根管形成したときのProTaper Ni-Ti製ファイルの相対性能を評価することを本研究の目的とした。

方法：ヒト上顎大臼歯を、解像度36μmのマイクロCTを用いて、ProTaperによる根管形成前後にスキャンした。根管を三次元的に再構築し、そして体積、表面積、厚み（直径）、根管の変位（トランスポーテーション）、および形成面で評価した。根管体積の中央値に基づいて、根管を、太い根管と狭窄根管に分類した。比較は、反復測定分散分析およびScheffe's post hoc testを用いて、広い根管と狭窄根管だけでなく、頬側近心根、遠心頬側根、および口蓋根という根管のタイプ間でも比較した。

結果：根管の体積と表面積は、近心頬側根、遠心頬側根、口蓋根において有意に同様な増加を示しており、そして著しい根管形成の失敗は稀であった。根尖の根管径と根尖から5mm歯冠側離れた部位の根管径では、近心頬側根において0.38mmから0.65mmへ、遠心頬側根において0.42mmから0.66mmへ、そして口蓋根において0.57mmから0.79mmへ、それぞれ増加していた。根尖部根管の変位（トランスポーテーション）は、根管のタイプとは無関係に0.02mmから0.4mmの変位量を示し、太い根管は狭窄根管と比べて未形成領域の割合が有意に高かった（P＜0.05）。

結論：上顎大臼歯の根管は、*in vitro*において、大きな失敗なくProTaperファイルを用いて根管形成可能であった。これらのProTaper器具は、幼若永久歯のような太い根管よりも、むしろ狭窄した根管の形成に用いたほうがより効果的かもしれない。

（Int Endod J 2003；36（2）：86-92.）

AIM: To evaluate the relative performance of ProTaper nickel-titanium (Ni-Ti) instruments shaping root canals of varying preoperative canal geometry.

METHODOLOGY: Extracted human maxillary molars were scanned, before and after shaping with ProTaper, employing micro computed tomography (muCT) at a resolution of 36 mum. Canals were three-dimensionally reconstructed and evaluated for volume, surface area, "thickness" (diameter), canal transportation and prepared surface. Based on median canal volume, canals were divided into "wide" and "constricted" groups. Comparisons were made between mesiobuccal (mb), distobuccal (db) and palatal(p), as well as "wide" and "constricted" canals, using repeated-measures anova and Scheffé posthoc tests.

RESULTS: Volume and surface area increased significantly and similarly in mb, db and p canals, and gross preparation errors were found infrequently. Root canal diameters, 5mm coronal to the apex, increased from 0.38 to 0.65 mm 0.42 to 0.66 mm and 0.57 to 0.79 mm for mb, db and p canals, respectively. Apical canal transportation ranged from 0.02 to 0.40 mm and was independent of canal type; "wide" canals had a significantly higher (P<0.05) proportion of unprepared surfaces than "constricted" canals.

CONCLUSIONS: Canals in maxillary molars were prepared *in vitro* using ProTaper instruments without major procedural errors. These instruments may be more effective in shaping narrow canals than wider, immature ones.

5 *Rotary nickel-titanium instruments*

引用数 **9**位

Dynamic and cyclic fatigue of engine-driven rotary nickel-titanium endodontic instruments.

歯内療法用 Ni-Ti 製ロータリーエンジンファイルの動的疲労と繰り返し疲労

Haïkel Y, Serfaty R, Bateman G, Senger B, Allemann C.

　エンジン駆動型 Ni-Ti 製ファイルを試験するための適切な基準がないことは、あらゆる領域におけるこれら器具のさらなる研究の必要性を意味する。本研究は、3種のエンジン駆動型 Ni-Ti 製ロータリー歯内療法用ファイル（Profile、Hero、および Quantec）を検索対象とし、根管形成中に器具に影響を与えた曲率半径に関する動的破壊時間を評価し、さらに破折が生じたときのサイズとテーパーに基づいたファイル径とそのときの破折様相も評価した。それぞれのファイル群と曲率半径にそれぞれのサイズとテーパーが行きわたるように10本のファイルを無作為に選び、計600本のファイルとした。ファイルは毎分350回転の速度で、模擬根管として焼戻しして処理された綱曲線金型に挿入した。5mm と10mm の2種類の曲率半径を適用した。すべてのファイルの破折までに要する時間を記録し、それぞれのファイルの破折面を電子顕微鏡で分析した。曲率半径が、ファイルの破折抵抗性を決定するもっとも有意な要因であるとわかった。曲率半径が小さくなるにつれて、破折までに要する時間は短くなった。ファイルのテーパーも破折時間の決定に重要であるとわかった。直径が大きくなるほど、破折に要する時間は短くなった。すべてのケースで、破折は、延性特性によるものであった。こうして、ファイル破折の主原因は繰り返し疲労破折であることがわかり、この分野におけるさらなる解析や基準の設置が必要であることがわかった。

（J Endod 1999；25（6）：434-440.）

The absence of adequate testing standards for engine-driven nickel-titanium (NiTi) instruments necessitates further study of these instruments in all areas. This study examined three groups of engine-driven rotary NiTi endodontic instruments (Profile, Hero, and Quantec) and assessed the times for dynamic fracture in relation to the radius of curvature to which the instruments were subjected during preparation, with the instrument diameter determined by size and taper and the mode by which the fracture occurred. Ten instruments were randomly selected representing each size and taper for each group and for each radius of curvature: 600 in total. The instruments were rotated at 350 rpm and introduced into a tempered steel curve that simulated a canal. Two radii of curvature of canals were used: 5 and 10 mm. Time at fracture was noted for all files, and the fracture faces of each file were analyzed with scanning electron microscopy. Radius of curvature was found to be the most significant factor in determining the fatigue resistance of the files. As radius of curvature decreased, fracture time decreased. Taper of files was found to be significant in determining fracture time. As diameter increased, fracture time decreased. In all cases, fracture was found to be of a ductile nature, thus implicating cyclic fatigue as a major cause of failure and necessitating further analyses and setting of standards in this area.

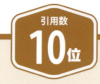

Rotary NiTi instrument fracture and its consequences.

Ni-Ti 製ロータリーファイルの破折とその原因

Parashos P, Messer HH.

　歯内療法器具の破折は、普段の日常診療に多大な支障をきたす処置上の問題である。Ni-Ti 製ロータリーファイルの出現により、このファイル破折という問題は、おそらく Ni-Ti という大きな技術的進歩を採用するにあたり、相当な障害として際立ってくるであろう。破折の発生頻度を最小限にするため、Ni-Ti 製合金破損のメカニズムを理解しようとする数多くの研究が行われている。このことは、器具のデザイン、プロトコル、および製造法の点において変化をもたらしている。加えて、経験、テクニック、そして能力という術者に関する要因にも影響を与えているようにみえる。本稿で提示する論文の評価から、われわれは、この偶発症の予防と対処に関する臨床指針を導くこととする。

（J Endod 2006；32(11)：1031-1043.）

The fracture of endodontic instruments is a procedural problem creating a major obstacle to normally routine therapy. With the advent of rotary nickel-titanium (NiTi) instruments this issue seems to have assumed such prominence as to be a considerable hindrance to the adoption of this major technical advancement. Considerable research has been undertaken to understand the mechanisms of failure of NiTi alloy to minimize its occurrence. This has led to changes in instrument design, instrumentation protocols, and manufacturing methods. In addition, factors related to clinician experience, technique, and competence have been shown to be influential. From an assessment of the literature presented. we derive clinical recommendations concerning prevention and management of this complication.

[5] Rotary nickel-titanium instruments

Shaping ability of ProFile.04 Taper Series 29 rotary nickel-titanium instruments in simulated root canals. Part 1.

ProFile.04 Series29 Ni-Ti 製ロータリーファイルの模擬根管における根管形成能。パート1

Thompson SA, Dummer PM.

　本研究の目的は、ProFile.04 Series29 Ni-Ti 製ロータリーファイルの根管形成能を測定することであった。湾曲の角度と位置の異なる4種類の形状を有するように作成された合計40の模擬根管を、ステップダウン形成を用いて ProFile ファイルで根管形成した。この2部構成レポートの第1部では、根管形成時間、ファイルの破損、根管の閉塞、根管長の短縮化および三次元的な形成後の根管形態に関するこのファイルの効率を述べる。根管形成に要した時間は根管形状による有意な影響は受けなかった。ファイルの破折は生じなかったが、総計52本のファイルが変形していた。サイズ6のファイルがもっとも多数変形し、続いてファイルサイズ5、3、および4の順に変形の頻度が高かった。根管の形状はファイルの変形に有意な影響を与えなかった。いずれの根管もデブリーによる閉塞は生じておらず、そして（根管形成による）作業長の短縮化は平均0.5mm 以下であった。形成した根管の管腔内の様相は、ほとんどの根管において明確なアピカルストップ、滑らかな根管壁および見事に移行的なテーパーを呈していた。ProFile.04 Series29 Ni-Ti 製ロータリーファイルは速やかに根管形成し、そして見事な三次元的形状を根管に作成した。相当数のファイルが変形したが、本実験モデルの性質上、そして設計上の固有の欠点のために、この変形現象が起きたかどうかの明確化はできなかった。

(Int Endod J 1997 ; 30(1) : 1-7.)

The aim of this study was to determine the shaping ability of ProFile.04 Taper Series 29 nickel-titanium instruments in simulated canals. A total of 40 simulated root canals made up of four different shapes in terms of angle and position of curvature were prepared by ProFile instruments using a step-down approach. Part 1 of this two-part report describes the efficacy of the instruments in terms of preparation time, instrument failure, canal blockages, loss of canal length and three-dimensional canal form. The time necessary for canal preparation was not influenced significantly by canal shape. No instrument fractures occurred but a total of 52 instruments deformed. Size 6 instruments deformed the most followed by sizes 5, 3 and 4. Canal shape did not influence significantly instrument deformation. None of the canals became blocked with debris and loss of working distance was on average 0.5 mm or less. Intracanal impressions of canal form demonstrated that most canals had definite apical stops, smooth canal walls and good flow and taper. Under the conditions of this study, ProFile.04 Taper Series 29 rotary nickel-titanium instruments prepared simulated canals rapidly and created good three-dimensional form. A substantial number of instruments deformed but it was not possible to determine whether this phenomenon occurred because of the nature of the experimental model or through an inherent design weakness in the instruments.

エンドのための重要20キーワード

6 Curved root canals
湾曲根管

通常の歯内療法においては、細いファイルから太いファイルへと順次、根尖部を拡大後、最終ファイルの号数と同じサイズのガッタパーチャポイントを充填するという手法が確立されている。しかしこの手法は、ときとして、根尖部における apical transportation が生じやすく、とくに、その apical transportation は湾曲根管において顕著になる。その問題点を解決するために、以前よりスチール製ファイルによる種々の根管形成法が報告されている。Ni-Ti 製ファイルによる根管形成は、スチール製ファイルによる形成と比較して、切削効率や作業時間の短縮とともに、根管追従性に優れていると多数の報告がしており、Ni-Ti 製ファイルを用いた湾曲根管の根管形成に対する報告も多数ある。

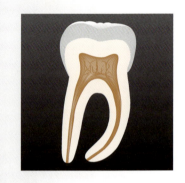

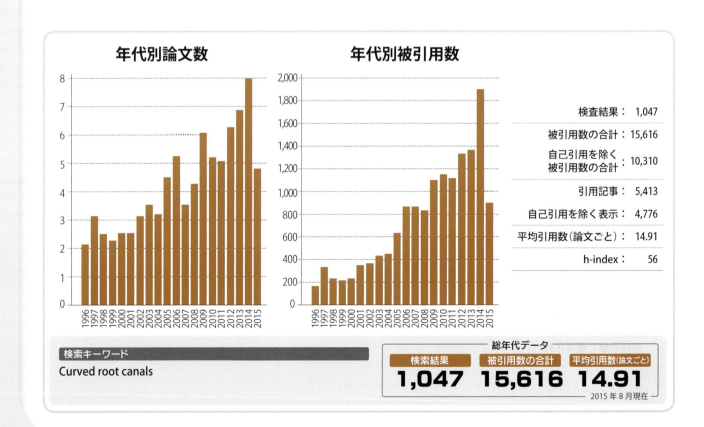

検索キーワード：Curved root canals

検査結果	1,047
被引用数の合計	15,616
自己引用を除く被引用数の合計	10,310
引用記事	5,413
自己引用を除く表示	4,776
平均引用数（論文ごと）	14.91
h-index	56

総年代データ
- 検索結果：1,047
- 被引用数の合計：15,616
- 平均引用数（論文ごと）：14.91

2015年8月現在

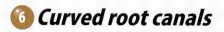

トムソン・ロイターが選んだベスト12論文

	タイトル・和訳	2011年	2012年	2013年	2014年	合計引用数
引用数 1位	Schneider SW. A comparison of canal preparations in straight and curved root canals. Oral Surg Oral Med Oral Pathol 1971；32(2)：271-275. 直線根管と湾曲根管における根管形成の比較 **本項に和訳あり**	35	40	28	49	565
引用数 2位	Pruett JP, Clement DJ, Carnes DL Jr. Cyclic fatigue testing of nickel-titanium endodontic instruments. J Endod 1997；23(2)：77-85. 根管形成用 Ni-Ti 製ファイルの繰り返し疲労試験 **本項に和訳あり**	25	36	26	27	360
引用数 3位	Peters OA. Current challenges and concepts in the preparation of root canal systems：a review. J Endod 2004；30(8)：559-567. 根管系の形成における現在の挑戦とコンセプト：総説論文 **チャプター15に和訳あり**	28	29	30	41	275
引用数 4位	Sattapan B, Nervo GJ, Palamara JE, Messer HH. Defects in rotary nickel-titanium files after clinical use. J Endod 2000；26(3)：161-165. 臨床使用後の Ni-Ti 製ロータリーファイル欠損 **本項に和訳あり**	20	22	22	37	243
引用数 5位	Roane JB, Sabala CL, Duncanson MG Jr. The "balanced force" concept for instrumentation of curved canals. J Endod 1985；11(5)：203-211. 湾曲根管を根管形成するためのバランスドフォースのコンセプト **本項に和訳あり**	4	9	8	15	237
引用数 6位	Reeh ES, Messer HH, Douglas WH. Reduction in tooth stiffness as a result of endodontic and restorative procedures. J Endod 1989；15(11)：512-516. 歯内療法操作および修復処置の結果生じる歯の剛性の減弱	14	8	14	20	193
引用数 7位	Thompson SA. An overview of nickel-titanium alloys used in dentistry. Int Endod J 2000；33(4)：297-310. 歯科治療で使用される Ni-Ti 製合金の概要	14	19	16	20	168

トムソン・ロイターが選んだベスト12論文

	タイトル・和訳	2011年	2012年	2013年	2014年	合計引用数
引用数 8位	Siqueira JF Jr, Rôças IN. Polymerase chain reaction-based analysis of microorganisms associated with failed endodontic treatment. Oral Surg Oral Med Oral Pathol Oral Radiol Endod 2004；97（1）：85-94. 歯内療法失敗治療に関与する細菌のポリメラーゼ連鎖反応（PCR）解析	18	10	11	20	162
引用数 9位	Haïkel Y, Serfaty R, Bateman G, Senger B, Allemann C. Dynamic and cyclic fatigue of engine-driven rotary nickel-titanium endodontic instruments. J Endod 1999；25（6）：434-440. 歯内療法用 Ni-Ti 製ロータリーエンジンファイルの動的疲労と繰り返し疲労 **チャプター5に和訳あり**	11	8	12	9	142
引用数 10位	Esposito PT, Cunningham CJ. A comparison of canal preparation with nickel-titanium and stainless steel instruments. J Endod 1995；21（4）：173-176. Ni-Ti 製ファイルとステンレススチール製ファイルを使用した根管形成の比較	3	2	5	4	131
引用数 11位	Abou-Rass M, Frank AL, Glick DH. The anticurvature filing method to prepare the curved root canal. J Am Dent Assoc 1980；101（5）：792-794. 湾曲根管を形成するための Anti-curvature ファイル法	3	3	6	10	126
引用数 12位	Wu MK, Wesselink PR. A primary observation on the preparation and obturation of oval canals. Int Endod J 2001；4（2）：137-141. 楕円形根管の根管形成と根管充填の一次観察	10	10	8	9	118

Curved root canals

A comparison of canal preparations in straight and curved root canals.

直線根管と湾曲根管における根管形成の比較

Schneider SW.

ヒト単根永久歯の抜去歯を歯根の湾曲度に応じて分類した。手用器具を用いて根管形成し、根管を断面観察したところ、まっすぐな根管では湾曲根管に比べ、より容易に円形状に根管形成されていた。

（Oral Surg Oral Med Oral Pathol 1971；32（2）：271-275.）

Extracted human single-rooted permanent teeth were classified according to degree of root curvature. Following hand instrumentation of the root canals, an examination of cross sections revealed that straight canals were much more readily prepared round than were curved canals.

Cyclic fatigue testing of nickel-titanium endodontic instruments.

根管形成用 Ni-Ti 製ファイルの繰り返し疲労試験

Pruett JP, Clement DJ, Carnes DL Jr.

　ライトスピードファイル破折時における根管の湾曲と動作速度の影響を測定することから、根管形成用 Ni-Ti 製ロータリーエンジン器具の繰り返し疲労を検索した。湾曲角度と湾曲半径の両方を測定可能な新しい根管湾曲度評価法が導入された。湾曲角度30°、45°、および60°、そして湾曲半径 2 mm もしくは 5 mm という仕様の 6 種のステンレススチール製のガイド管で、湾曲根管を実験的に再現した。30号と40号のライトスピードファイルは、ガイドチューブに挿入され、そして Mangtrol トルクスピード計測計の口金にファイルヘッドを固定した。模擬操作荷重は10 g/cm を適用した。ファイルは、破折するまで750、1,300、あるいは2,000rpm の回転数で試験装置のなかを自由に回転操作可能であった。破折時の破壊寿命を測定した。破壊寿命は回転数の影響を受けなかった。ファイルは先端部で破折せずに、むしろガイドチューブの湾曲中心点に相当するファイル柄の最大屈曲点で破折した。同一実験条件下では、30号ファイルと比べてより太い40号ファイルのほうが、有意に破壊寿命が短かった。湾曲半径が 5 mm から 2 mm に減少した場合、そして湾曲度が30°以上の場合も同様に破壊寿命が短くなることが、多変量解析の結果より示された（$P < 0.05$、power $= 0.9$）。走査型電子顕微鏡を用いた評価は疲労破折の様式として延性破折を示した。これらの結果から、根管形成用 Ni-Ti 製ロータリーエンジン器具破折の目安としては、動作速度よりも湾曲半径、湾曲角度、および器具サイズが重要であることがわかった。本研究は、周期的疲労破壊の技術コンセプトを支持するものであり、そして Ni-Ti 製ロータリーファイルの規格化破壊試験を行うためには、湾曲状態において動的なファイル操作を考慮して行うべきであると示唆している。本研究結果は、根管形成評価の際には、ひとつの独立変数として湾曲半径の影響を考慮すべきであることを示唆した。

(J Endod 1997；23（2）：77-85.)

Cyclic fatigue of nickel-titanium, engine-driven instruments was studied by determining the effect of canal curvature and operating speed on the breakage of Lightspeed instruments. A new method of canal curvature evaluation that addressed both angle and abruptness of curvature was introduced. Canal curvature was simulated by constructing six curved stainless-steel guide tubes with angles of curvature of 30, 45, or 60 degrees, and radii of curvature of 2 or 5mm. Size #30 and #40 Light-speed instruments were placed through the guide tubes and the heads secured in the collet of a Mangtrol Dynamometer. A simulated operating load of 10 g-cm was applied. Instruments were able to rotate freely in the test apparatus at speeds of 750, 1,300, or 2,000rpm until separation occurred. Cycles to failure were determined. Cycles to failure were not affected by rpm. Instruments did not separate at the head, but rather at the point of maximum flexure of the shaft, corresponding to the midpoint of curvature within the guide tube. The instruments with larger diameter shafts, #40, failed after significantly fewer cycles than did #30 instruments under identical test conditions. Multivariable analysis of variance indicated that cycles to failure significantly decreased as the radius of curvature decreased from 5mm to 2mm and as the angle of curvature increased greater than 30 degrees($p<0.05$, power$=0.9$). Scanning electron microscopic evaluation revealed ductile fracture as the fatigue failure mode. These results indicate that, for nickel-titanium, engine-driven rotary instruments, the radius of curvature, angle of curvature, and instrument size are more important than operating speed for predicting separation. This study supports engineering concepts of cyclic fatigue failure and suggests that standardized fatigue tests of nickel-titanium rotary instruments should include dynamic operation in a flexed state. The results also suggest that the effect of the radius of curvature as an independent variable should be considered when evaluating studies of root canal instrumentation.

Curved root canals

Defects in rotary nickel-titanium files after clinical use.

臨床使用後の Ni-Ti 製ロータリーファイル欠損

Sattapan B, Nervo GJ, Palamara JE, Messer HH.

　本研究の目的は、日常臨床に使用された後の Ni-Ti 製ロータリーファイルの欠損様式と欠損頻度について分析し、そしてその欠損理由を明らかにすることである。6 か月以上歯内療法専門医が使用して破棄したファイルのすべて（総本数378本、Quantec Series 2000）を分析した。ほぼ半数のファイルには、肉眼で識別可能な欠損が観察され、21%のファイルが破折しており、そして28%のファイルには破折以外の欠損が認められた。破折ファイルは観察された欠損の特徴により 2 つのグループに分類された。ねじれ破折は全破折ファイル中55.7%に、一方、屈曲疲労は44.3%に生じていた。以上の結果は、ねじれ破折は、根管形成中に根尖方向へ力をかけすぎたため、屈曲疲労よりもさらに頻繁に起き、そして湾曲根管で使用した結果起きることを示唆していた。

（J Endod 2000；26（3）：161-165.）

The purpose of this study was to analyze the type and frequency of defects in nickel-titanium rotary endodontic files after routine clinical use, and to draw conclusions regarding the reasons for failure. All of the files (total:378, Quantec Series 2000) discarded after normal use from a specialist endodontic practice over 6 months were analyzed. Almost 50% of the files showed some visible defect; 21% were fractured and 28% showed other defects without fracture. Fractured files could be divided into two groups according to the characteristics of the defects observed. Torsional fracture occurred in 55.7% of all fractured files, whereas flexural fatigue occurred in 44.3%. The results indicated that torsional failure, which may be caused by using too much apical force during instrumentation, occurred more frequently than flexural fatigue, which may result from use in curved canals.

The "balanced force" concept for instrumentation of curved canals.

湾曲根管を根管形成するための バランスドフォースのコンセプト

Roane JB, Sabala CL, Duncanson MG Jr.

　根管の湾曲はつねに根管形成をややこしいものにしている。そこで12年以上の試行錯誤の実験から開発した"バランスドフォースのコンセプト"を、湾曲の影響を克服するための手段として提案する。このコンセプトは根管の湾曲に関連して生じる望ましからざる過剰切削を制御可能な力の大きさを用いている。正回転は基準となる力の大きさを維持する手段となり、そして逆方向へ回転することにより術者による有限制御が与えられる。コンセプトの各ステップを、図表評価、数理計算、曲げモーメント、研究用根管、薄切歯、および臨床エックス線写真として記録して本論文に示した。そのコンセプトは、新設計のKファイルを導入することで、実現可能となる。

（J Endod 1985；11（5）：203-211.）

Canal curvature has always introduced complexity into canal preparation. The "balanced force concept", developed by trial and error experimentation over the past 12yr, is proposed as a means of overcoming the curvature influence. Its concepts use force magnitudes in order to create control over undesirable cutting associated with canal curvature. Rotation is promoted as the means for maintaining magnitude as a control and counterclockwise direction of rotation provides finite operator control. Diagrammatic evaluations, mathematical calculations, bending moments, test canals, sectioned teeth, and clinical radiographs are presented to document each step of the concept. The concept comes to fruition with the introduction of a new K-type file design.

エンドのための重要20キーワード

7 Root canal transportation

根管の移動（偏位）

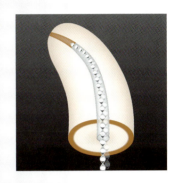

　湾曲根管を根管形成する際、ファイル等の器具の有する剛性のため、湾曲の外湾部が選択的に切削された結果、根管の中心点に偏位が生じる。これらの偏位はRoot canal transportationと呼ばれる。この偏位が、過度になると、根管は直線化し、レッジ形成、ZIP形成などが生じる。そのため、根管原型を保持した根管形成を維持するための研究が、これまでも数多くなされている。

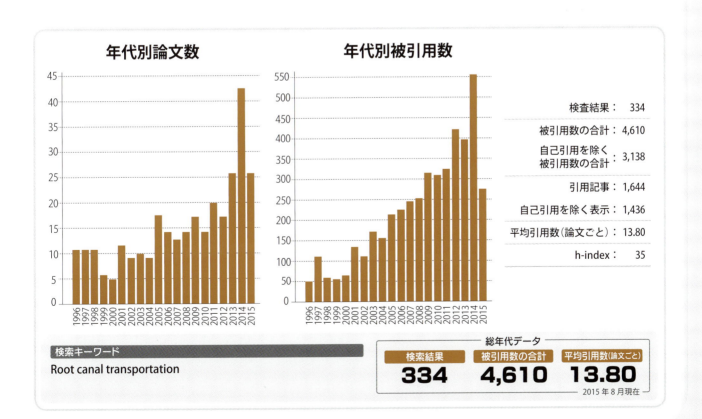

年代別論文数　　年代別被引用数

検査結果： 334
被引用数の合計： 4,610
自己引用を除く被引用数の合計： 3,138
引用記事： 1,644
自己引用を除く表示： 1,436
平均引用数（論文ごと）： 13.80
h-index： 35

検索キーワード
Root canal transportation

総年代データ
検索結果 334　被引用数の合計 4,610　平均引用数（論文ごと） 13.80

2015年8月現在

トムソン・ロイターが選んだベスト**12**論文

	タイトル・和訳	2011年	2012年	2013年	2014年	合計引用数
引用数 1位	Glossen CR, Haller RH, Dove SB, del Rio CE. A comparison of root canal preparations using Ni-Ti hand, Ni-Ti engine-driven, and K-Flex endodontic instruments. J Endod 1995；21（3）：146-151. 手用Ni-Ti製ファイル、エンジン駆動型Ni-Ti製ファイルおよびK-Flexファイルを用いた根管形成の比較 **本項に和訳あり**	8	15	13	17	252
引用数 2位	Peters OA, Schönenberger K, Laib A. Effects of four Ni-Ti preparation techniques on root canal geometry assessed by micro computed tomography. Int Endod J 2001；34（3）：221-230. マイクロCTにより評価された4種のNi-Ti製根管形成手技の根管形態に対する影響 **本項に和訳あり**	17	23	21	29	189
引用数 3位	Peters OA, Peters CI, Schönenberger K, Barbakow F. ProTaper rotary root canal preparation：effects of canal anatomy on final shape analysed by micro CT. Int Endod J 2003；36（2）：86-92. ProTaperロータリーファイルによる根管形成：最終形成が根管解剖に及ぼす影響についてのマイクロCTによる評価 **チャプター5に和訳あり**	15	21	8	16	142
引用数 4位	Peters OA, Laib A, Göhring TN, Barbakow F. Changes in root canal geometry after preparation assessed by high-resolution computed tomography. J Endod 2001；27（1）：1-6. 高解像度CTにより評価された根管形成後の根管形態の変化 **本項に和訳あり**	13	12	13	10	125
引用数 5位	Nielsen RB, Alyassin AM, Peters DD, Carnes DL, Lancaster J. Micro-computed tomography：an advanced system for detailed endodontic research. J Endod 1995；21（11）：561-568. マイクロCT：詳細な歯内療法学の研究のための先進システム	6	7	4	8	96
引用数 6位	Gambill JM, Alder M, del Rio CE. Comparison of nickel-titanium and stainless steel hand-file instrumentation using computed tomography. J Endod 1996；22（7）：369-375. CTを用いたNi-Ti製とステンレススチール製手用ファイルの根管形成の比較	5	9	7	10	95

Root canal transportation

トムソン・ロイターが選んだベスト12論文

	タイトル・和訳	2011年	2012年	2013年	2014年	合計引用数
引用数 7位	Short JA, Morgan LA, Baumgartner JC. A comparison of canal centering ability of four instrumentation techniques. J Endod 1997；23（8）：503-507. 4種の根管形成手技の根管中心保持能力の比較 **本項に和訳あり**	3	2	7	10	91
引用数 8位	Bergmans L, Van Cleynenbreugel J, Wevers M, Lambrechts P. A methodology for quantitative evaluation of root canal instrumentation using microcomputed tomography. Int Endod J 2001；34（5）：390-398. マイクロCTを用いた根管形成の定量評価法	5	9	4	3	79
引用数 9位	Bergmans L, Van Cleynenbreugel J, Wevers M, Lambrechts P. Mechanical root canal preparation with NiTi rotary instruments：rationale, performance and safety. Status report for the American Journal of Dentistry. Am J Dent 2001；14（5）：324-333. Ni-Ti製ロータリーファイルによる機械的根管形成。American Journal of Dentistryにおける進捗レポート	4	6	5	16	71
引用数 10位	Versümer J, Hülsmann M, Schäfers F. A comparative study of root canal preparation using Profile .04 and Lightspeed rotary Ni-Ti instruments. Int Endod J 2002；35（1）：37-46. ProFile .04とLightspeedロータリーファイルを用いた根管形成の比較試験	4	1	4	3	70
引用数 11位	Thompson SA, Dummer PM. Shaping ability of ProFile.04 Taper Series 29 rotary nickel-titanium instruments in simulated root canals. Part 2. Int Endod J 1997；30（1）：8-15. ProFile.04 Series29 NI-Ti製ロータリーファイルの模擬根管における根管形成能。パート2	3	1	2	1	67
引用数 12位	Bergmans L, Van Cleynenbreugel J, Beullens M, Wevers M, Van Meerbeek B, Lambrechts P. Progressive versus constant tapered shaft design using NiTi rotary instruments. Int Endod J 2003；36（4）：288-295. Ni-Ti製ロータリーファイルの先進的テーパーシャフトデザインVS 一定のテーパーシャフトデザイン	10	9	3	3	65

A comparison of root canal preparations using Ni-Ti hand, Ni-Ti engine-driven, and K-Flex endodontic instruments.

手用 Ni-Ti 製ファイル、エンジン駆動型 Ni-Ti 製ファイルおよび K-Flex ファイルを用いた根管形成の比較

Glossen CR, Haller RH, Dove SB, del Rio CE.

　本研究は、手用 Ni-Ti 製ファイル、エンジン駆動型 Ni-Ti 製ファイル、および手用ステンレススチール製ファイルによる根管形成を比較するために駆動型改良型 Bramante 法とデジタル減算ソフトウェアを用いた。60根のヒト下顎大臼歯抜去歯の近心根を、無作為に5群に分類した。歯根は、透明レジンに包埋した後、根尖部と根中央部において横断した。実験群 A においては、K-Flex ファイルを用いターンアンドプル（turn and pull）法で根管を形成した。実験群 B においては、手用 Ni-Ti 製ファイル（Mity）を用い実験群 A と同様にターンアンドプル（turn and pull）法で根管形成した。実験群 C はエンジン駆動型 Ni-Ti 製ファイル（NT Sensor）で形成した。実験群 D は手用 Ni-Ti 製ファイル（Ni-Ti Canal Master "U"）で形成した。実験群 E はエンジン駆動型 Ni-Ti 製ファイル（Lightspeed）で形成した。根管形成前のデジタル画像と根管形成後のデジタル画像が比較された。エンジン駆動型 Ni-Ti 製ファイル（NT Sensor、Lightspeed）および手用 Ni-Ti 製ファイル（Ni-Ti Canal Master"U"）は、K-Flex や Mity ファイルより、根管の偏位（トランスポーテーション）を有意に小さく（$P<0.05$）、根管中心を有意に保持し（$P<0.05$）、象牙質切削量も有意に少なく（$P<0.05$）、そしてより円形に近く根管形成していた。NT Sensor と Lightspeed によるエンジン駆動を用いた根管形成は、手用ファイルより有意に早く根管形成できた（$P<0.05$）。

（J Endod 1995；21（3）：146-151.）

This study used a modified Bramante technique and new digital subtraction software to compare root canals prepared by nickel-titanium (Ni-Ti) hand, Ni-Ti engine-driven, and stainless steel hand endodontic instruments. Sixty mesial canals of extracted human mandibular molars were randomly divided into five groups. The roots were embedded in clear resin and cross-sectioned in the apical and mid-root areas. In group A, canals were instrumented using a quarter turn/pull technique with K-Flex files. In group B, canals were prepared with Ni-Ti hand files (Mity files) using the same technique as in group A. Group C was prepared with NT Sensor engine-driven files. Group D canals were prepared with Ni-Ti Canal Master "U" hand instruments. Group E was prepared with engine-driven Ni-Ti Lightspeed instruments. Digitized images of the uninstrumented canals were compared with images of the instrumented canals. Engine-driven Ni-Ti instruments (Lightspeed and NT Sensor file) and hand instrumentation with the Canal Master "U" caused significantly less canal transportation ($p<0.05$), remained more centered in the canal ($p<0.05$), removed less dentin ($p<0.05$), and produced rounder canal preparations than K-Flex and Mity files. Engine instrumentation with Lightspeed and NT Sensor file was significantly faster than hand instrumentation ($p<0.05$).

Root canal transportation

Effects of four Ni-Ti preparation techniques on root canal geometry assessed by micro computed tomography.

マイクロCTにより評価された4種のNi-Ti製根管形成手技の根管形態に対する影響

Peters OA, Schönenberger K, Laib A.

目的：本研究は、ヒト上顎大臼歯抜去歯から三次元的に再現された根管を用い、4つの根管形成手技の効果を根管の体積と表面積に対して比較した。加えて、マイクロCTデータを、4種の根管形成手技に関する形態計測のパラメータ描写のために使用した。

方法：マイクロCTスキャナは上顎大臼歯抜去歯の根管解析に用いられた。Ni-Ti製Kファイル、Lightspeedファイル、ProFile.04およびGTロータリーファイルを用いた根管形成前と後に、標本をそれぞれスキャンした。象牙質削除量、根管の直線化、未形成領域の割合、そして根管偏位の差を、特別に開発したソフトを用いて計算した。

結果：根管形成により、根管の体積と表面積は増大した。形成された根管は、未形成の根管と比べて、有意な円形化、径の増大化、および直線化を示していた。しかしながら、どの根管形成テクニックを用いても、根管表面積の35%以上がいまだ形成されないまま残っていた。検索した3種の根管形態間に有意差が認められた一方で、根管形成手技による差はほとんど認められなかった。

結論：マイクロCTシステム解析では、4種の根管形成手技に差はほとんど認められなかった。対照的に、根管形態の相違による多大な影響が示された。根管形成の生体力学的側面について十分に理解するためには、三次元的解析法を用いたさらなる研究が必要となる。

（Int Endod J 2001；34（3）：221-230.）

AIM: The aim of this study was to compare the effects of four preparation techniques on canal volume and surface area using three-dimensionally reconstructed root canals in extracted human maxillary molars. In addition, micro CT data was used to describe morphometric parameters related to the four preparation techniques.
METHODOLOGY: A micro computed tomography scanner was used to analyse root canals in extracted maxillary molars. Specimens were scanned before and after canals were prepared using Ni-Ti-K-Files, Lightspeed instruments, ProFile.04 and GT rotary instruments. Differences in dentine volume removed, canal straightening, the proportion of unchanged area and canal transportation were calculated using specially developed software.
RESULTS: Instrumentation of canals increased volume and surface area. Prepared canals were significantly more rounded, had greater diameters and were straighter than unprepared canals. However, all instrumentation techniques left 35% or more of the canals' surface area unchanged. Whilst there were significant differences between the three canal types investigated, very few differences were found with respect to instrument types.
CONCLUSIONS: Within the limitations of the micro CT system, there were few differences between the four canal instrumentation techniques used. By contrast, a strong impact of variations of canal anatomy was demonstrated. Further studies with 3D-techniques are required to fully understand the biomechanical aspects of root canal preparation.

Changes in root canal geometry after preparation assessed by high-resolution computed tomography.

高解像度 CT により評価された根管形成後の根管形態の変化

Peters OA, Laib A, Göhring TN, Barbakow F.

　根管の解剖学的形態は根管形成中に変化し、これらの変化は用いる術式によりおそらく異なってくるであろう。そうした変化を根管形成前後の横断面を計測することにより in vitro において研究した。今回のこの研究では、根管形成後の根管網における変化を評価するために、非破壊的に評価可能な高解像度 CT を用いた。マイクロ CT スキャナ（空間分解能 cubic resolution 34ミクロン）を抜去歯6歯における18根管の解析のために用いた。根管は、K ファイル、Lightspeed ファイル、および ProFile .04ロータリーファイルを用いた根管形成の術前・術後においてそれぞれスキャンされた。特別な据え付け装置を用いることで、根管形成後の標本を正確に再配置し、スキャンすることが可能であった。それぞれの根管の形成前後の表面積（deltaA in mm^2）と体積（deltaV in mm^3）の相違は特注のソフトウェアを用いて計算された。deltaV は、1.61±0.7の平均で、値の範囲は0.64から2.86であり、一方、deltaA は4.16±2.63の平均で、値の範囲は0.72から9.66であった。K ファイル、Lightspeed ファイル、および ProFile .04ロータリーファイルの deltaV と deltaA の平均値は、それぞれ deltaV 1.28±0.57、deltaA 2.58±1.83；deltaV 1.79±0.66、deltaA 4.86±2.53；deltaV 1.81±0.57、deltaA 5.31±2.98であった。根管の解剖学的形態と根管形成の影響は、さらに構造モデル指標（structure model index）と the Transportation of Centers of Mass を用いて解析された。本研究条件下では、術式それ自体よりも術前のいろいろな根管形状が、根管形成中の変化にさらに影響を及ぼしていた。したがって、根管の解剖学的形態に対する根管形成器具の影響を比較する研究では、術前の根管形状のディテールも考慮すべきであると考えられる。

（J Endod 2001；27(1)：1-6.）

Root canal morphology changes during canal preparation, and these changes may vary depending on the technique used. Such changes have been studied *in vitro* by measuring cross-sections of canals before and after preparation. This current study used nondestructive high-resolution scanning tomography to assess changes in the canals' paths after preparation. A microcomputed tomography scanner (cubic resolution 34microm) was used to analyze 18 canals in 6 extracted maxillary molars. Canals were scanned before and after preparation using either K-Files, Lightspeed, or ProFile .04 rotary instruments. A special mounting device enabled precise repositioning and scanning of the specimens after preparation. Differences in surface area (deltaA in mm^2) and volume (deltaV in mm^3) of each canal before and after preparation were calculated using custom-made software. deltaV ranged from 0.64 to 2.86, with a mean of 1.61+/-0.7, whereas deltaA varied from 0.72 to 9.66, with a mean of 4.16+/-2.63. Mean deltaV and deltaA for the K-File, ProFile, and Lightspeed groups were 1.28+/-0.57 and 2.58+/-1.83；1.79+/-0.66 and 4.86+/-2.53；and 1.81+/-0.57 and 5.31+/-2.98, respectively. Canal anatomy and the effects of preparation were further analyzed using the Structure Model Index and the Transportation of Centers of Mass. Under the conditions of this study variations in canal geometry before preparation had more influence on the changes during preparation than the techniques themselves. Consequently studies comparing the effects of root canal instruments on canal anatomy should also consider details of the preoperative canal geometry.

A comparison of canal centering ability of four instrumentation techniques.

4種の根管形成手技の根管中心保持能力の比較

Short JA, Morgan LA, Baumgartner JC.

　本研究の目的は根管偏位に対するファイルの影響を、手用ファイルと3種のエンジン駆動型 Ni-Ti 製ファイルで比較することである。独立した根管を有する成人下顎第一大臼歯の近心根を湾曲度と形態に基づき2根1組のペアにした。根管長を、根管口から根尖孔まで11mm の長さで規格化した。ペアにした歯の4根管を、3種のエンジン駆動型 Ni-Ti 製ファイル Profile、Lightspeed、McXIM、あるいは手用 Flex-R ファイルのいずれかで、無作為に割りふられた根管に対して、根管形成した。歯根を、改良型 Bramante 法を用い、備え付けた後、作業長から1mm、3mm、および5mm の位置で断面化した。すべての切片を、術前、30号で根管形成後、そして40号で最終的な根管形成を行った後にビデオ画像として録画した。画像から、根管領域の変化および根管形成各段階における中心点を、コンピュータ分析した。根管形成時間も記録された。データは ANOVA を用いて解析された。Ni-Ti 製ファイルシステムは、ステンレススチール製手用ファイルより根管の中心点をいっそう良好に保っていた。どの検索断面においても、3種の Ni-Ti 製ファイルシステム間に有意差は認められなかった。手用ファイルとの Ni-Ti 製による根管形成間の差は、30号より40号のファイルサイズでより顕著であった。40号付近のサイズのファイルで根管形成を行った場合、3種の Ni-Ti 製ファイルシステム間において、根管形成における有意差は認められなかった。

（J Endod 1997；23（8）：503-507.）

The purpose of this study was to compare three engine driven (nickel-titanium) NiTi instrument systems with hand files for their effect on canal transportation. Mesial roots of mature lower first molars with separate canals were paired on the basis of curvature and morphology. Canal lengths were standardized to 11mm from orifice to apical foramen. Profile, Lightspeed, McXIM, and Flex-R hand filing techniques respectively were randomly assigned to one of the four canals of each tooth pair. The roots were mounted and sectioned at 1mm, 3mm, and 5mm from working length using a modified Bramante technique. All sections were video imaged preoperatively after instrumentation to size #30 and after final instrumentation to size #40. The images were computer analyzed for changes in canal area and centering at each stage of instrumentation. Preparation time was also recorded. Data were analyzed using ANOVA. The NiTi systems remained better centered in the canal than stainless steel hand files. There were no significant differences among the NiTi systems at any level. The difference between hand filing and the NiTi techniques was more pronounced at size #40 than at size #30. The NiTi systems were all significantly faster than hand filing. No significant differences in preparation were found between the NiTi systems when canals were instrumented to the size nearest #40.

エンドのための重要20キーワード

8 Endodontic irrigation
根管洗浄

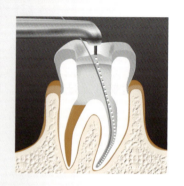

歯内療法を成功へ導く方法のひとつとして、十分な根管の化学的清掃が挙げられる。十分な根管洗浄と併用して実施される一連の根管拡大形成は、化学的機械的根管形成（Chemomechanical root canal preparation）といわれている。根管洗浄による化学的清掃は、機械的清掃では切削できなかった根管の非切削部位を洗浄によって補完できるため、非常に重要と考えられている。とりわけ次亜塩素酸ナトリウム（NaClO）は、抗菌作用と有機質溶解作用を有する強力な根管洗浄剤であり、次亜塩素酸ナトリウムに対する多数の研究が報告されている。

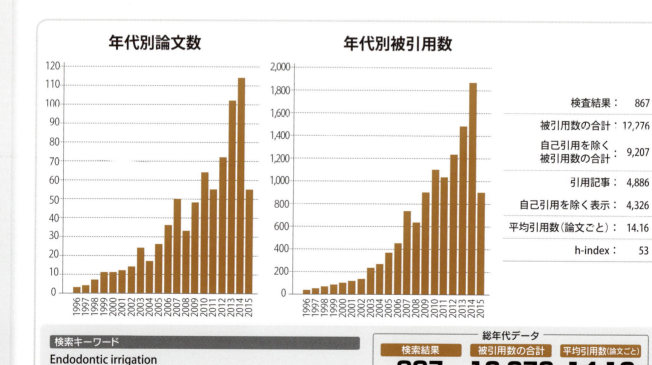

検索キーワード：Endodontic irrigation

検査結果： 867
被引用数の合計： 12,276
自己引用を除く被引用数の合計： 9,207
引用記事： 4,886
自己引用を除く表示： 4,326
平均引用数（論文ごと）： 14.16
h-index： 53

総年代データ
検索結果 867
被引用数の合計 12,276
平均引用数（論文ごと） 14.16

2015年8月現在

⑧ Endodontic irrigation

トムソン・ロイターが選んだベスト12論文

	タイトル・和訳	2011年	2012年	2013年	2014年	合計引用数
引用数 1位	Nair PN, Henry S, Cano V, Vera J. Microbial status of apical root canal system of human mandibular first molars with primary apical periodontitis after "one-visit" endodontic treatment. Oral Surg Oral Med Oral Pathol Oral Radiol Endod 2005；99（2）：231-252. 1回治療法を用いた歯内療法後の初発根尖病変を有するヒト下顎第一大臼歯根尖部根管系の細菌学的状態器 **本項に和訳あり**	31	27	27	27	256
引用数 2位	Byström A, Sundqvist G. Bacteriologic evaluation of the effect of 0.5 percent sodium hypochlorite in endodontic therapy. Oral Surg Oral Med Oral Pathol 1983；55（3）：307-312. 歯内療法における0.5％次亜塩素酸ナトリウムの効果に関する細菌学的評価 **本項に和訳あり**	15	20	6	13	252
引用数 3位	Spangberg L, Engström B, Langeland K. Biologic effects of dental materials. 3. Toxicity and antimicrobial effect of endodontic antiseptics *in vitro*. Oral Surg Oral Med Oral Pathol 1973；36（6）：856-871. 歯科材料の生物学的効果 3. *in vitro* における根管消毒剤の毒性と抗菌効果 **本項に和訳あり**	9	7	5	3	182
引用数 4位	Jeansonne MJ, White RR. A comparison of 2.0% chlorhexidine gluconate and 5.25% sodium hypochlorite as antimicrobial endodontic irrigants. J Endod 1994；20（6）：276-278. 抗菌性根管洗浄剤としての2％グルコン酸クロルヘキシジンと5.25％次亜塩素酸ナトリウムの比較 **本項に和訳あり**	10	9	6	15	177
引用数 5位	Shuping GB, Orstavik D, Sigurdsson A, Trope M. Reduction of intracanal bacteria using nickel-titanium rotary instrumentation and various medications. J Endod 2000；26（12）：751-755. Ni-Ti 製ロータリーファイルの根管形成とさまざまな薬物を使用した根管内細菌の減少 **本項に和訳あり**	11	14	10	20	160
引用数 6位	Calt S, Serper A. Time-dependent effects of EDTA on dentin structures. J Endod 2002；28（1）：17-19. 象牙質構造に及ぼす EDTA の時間依存性作用 **チャプター10に和訳あり**	14	13	18	10	149

エンドのための重要20キーワード（関連性の高い論文和訳）

トムソン・ロイターが選んだベスト**12**論文

	タイトル・和訳	2011年	2012年	2013年	2014年	合計引用数
引用数 7位	Gomes BP, Ferraz CC, Vianna ME, Berber VB, Teixeira FB, Souza-Filho FJ. In vitro antimicrobial activity of several concentrations of sodium hypochlorite and chlorhexidine gluconate in the elimination of Enterococcus faecalis. Int Endod J 2001 ; 34（6）: 424-428. Enterococcus faecalis 排除に関して次亜塩素酸とグルコン酸クロルヘキシジンをさまざまな濃度で使用した場合の in vitro における抗菌効果 チャプター9に和訳あり	13	14	16	14	148
引用数 8位	Peciuliene V, Reynaud AH, Balciuniene I, Haapasalo M. Isolation of yeasts and enteric bacteria in root-filled teeth with chronic apical periodontitis. Int Endod J 2001 ; 34（6）: 429-434. 慢性根尖性歯周炎を有する既根管充填歯における酵母菌と腸内細菌の分離	5	9	12	12	141
引用数 9位	White RR, Hays GL, Janer LR. Residual antimicrobial activity after canal irrigation with chlorhexidine. J Endod 1997 ; 23（4）: 229-231. クロルヘキシジンを用いた根管洗浄後の残存抗菌効果	14	6	7	7	128
引用数 10位	Sen BH, Wesselink PR, Türkün M. The smear layer : a phenomenon in root canal therapy. Int Endod J 1995 ; 28（3）: 141-148. スメアー層：根管治療における事象	5	6	7	7	126
引用数 11位	Card SJ, Sigurdsson A, Orstavik D, Trope M. The effectiveness of increased apical enlargement in reducing intracanal bacteria. J Endod 2002 ; 28(11) : 779-783. 根管内細菌の低減における根尖部での拡大を大きくしたときの有効性	4	9	10	11	122
引用数 12位	Peciuliene V, Balciuniene I, Eriksen HM, Haapasalo M. Isolation of Enterococcus faecalis in previously root-filled canals in a Lithuanian population. J Endod 2000 ; 26(10) : 593-595. リトアニア人の既充填根管における Enterococcus faecalis の分離	8	15	10	3	115

Endodontic irrigation

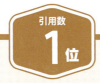

Microbial status of apical root canal system of human mandibular first molars with primary apical periodontitis after "one-visit" endodontic treatment.

１回治療法を用いた歯内療法後の初発根尖病変を有するヒト下顎第一大臼歯根尖部根管系の細菌学的状態

Nair PN, Henry S, Cano V, Vera J.

目的：歯内療法１回治療法治療後の初発根尖性歯周炎を有するヒト下顎第一大臼歯近心根の根尖部根管系の in vivo の根管内細菌状態を評価することを目的とした。根管内の残留感染は、光学顕微鏡と透過電子顕微鏡の相関視野観察により確認した。 **研究デザイン**：16歯の下顎第一大臼歯感染近心根管は、それぞれ歯内療法１回治療法による治療が行われた。近心頰側根はステンレス製手用ファイルを用いて、そして近心舌側根はNi-Ti製ロータリーシステムを用いて形成した。これらの根管を、根管形成中は5.25％次亜塩素酸ナトリウムを用いて根管洗浄し、10mLの17％エチレンジアミン４酢酸（EDTA）を用いて最終洗浄後、ガッタパーチャと酸化亜鉛ユージノールセメントを用いて根管充填した。その後、それぞれの歯の根尖部分をフラップ手術により取り除いた。サンプルは固定、脱灰、水平面で分割された後、樹脂包埋し、そして光学顕微鏡と透過電子顕微鏡の相関視野観察に供した後、評価された。 **結果**：根管形成、抗菌洗浄、そして根管充填した16歯の歯内治療歯のうち14歯において、根管内の残留感染が明らかとなった。細菌は、そのほとんどがバイオフィルムとして存在し、隔絶された凹み、形成後の主根管の憩室、根管イスムス、そして副根管に存在した。 **結論**：（１）下顎第一大臼歯歯根の根管系の解剖学的複雑性、（２）歯内療法１回治療法においては現在の器具や洗浄のみでは取り除くことのできない根管系の隔絶された場所におけるバイオフィルムとしての細菌叢の存在、という結果が明らかとなった。根管治療後の非常に良好な長期的予後を期待するために、バイオフィルムを破壊し、根尖部内の細菌や細菌関連物質を可能な限り低いレベルまで減少させて壊死感染根管歯の治療を行うためには、非抗菌的なあらゆる化学的機械的洗浄手段の徹底した使用が重要であることを、これらの所見は示している。

（Oral Surg Oral Med Oral Pathol Oral Radiol Endod 2005；99（２）：231-252.）

OBJECTIVE:To assess the *in vivo* intracanal microbial status of apical root canal system of mesial roots of human mandibular first molars with primary apical periodontitis immediately after one-visit endodontic treatment. The residual intracanal infection was confirmed by correlative light and transmission electron microscopy.
STUDY DESIGN:Sixteen diseased mesial roots of mandibular first molars were treated endodontically, each in one visit. Mesio-buccal canals were instrumented using stainless steel hand files and mesio-lingual canals with a nickel-titanium rotary system. The canals were irrigated with 5.25% sodium hypochlorite (NaOCl) during the instrumentation procedures, rinsed with 10mL of 17% ethylenediamine tetraacetic acid (EDTA), and obturated with gutta-percha and zinc oxide eugenol cement. Thereafter, the apical portion of the root of each tooth was removed by flap-surgery. The specimens were fixed, decalcified, subdivided in horizontal plane, embedded in plastic, processed ,and evaluated by correlative light and transmission electron microscopy.
RESULTS:Fourteen of the 16 endodontically treated teeth revealed residual intracanal infection after instrumentation, antimicrobial irrigation, and obturation. The microbes were located in inaccessible recesses and diverticula of instrumented main canals, the intercanal isthmus, and accessory canals, mostly as biofilms.
CONCLUSIONS:The results show (1) the anatomical complexity of the root canal system of mandibular first molar roots and (2) the organization of the flora as biofilms in inaccessible areas of the canal system that cannot be removed by contemporary instruments and irrigation alone in one-visit treatment. These findings demonstrate the importance of stringent application of all nonantibiotic chemo-mechanical measures to treat teeth with infected and necrotic root canals so as to disrupt the biofilms and reduce the intraradicular microbial load to the lowest possible level so as to expect a highly favorable long-term prognosis of the root canal treatment.

Bacteriologic evaluation of the effect of 0.5 percent sodium hypochlorite in endodontic therapy.

歯内療法における0.5％次亜塩素酸ナトリウムの効果に関する細菌学的評価

Byström A, Sundqvist G.

　15本の単根歯における根管洗浄剤としての0.5％次亜塩素酸ナトリウム溶液の抗菌効果を検索した。それぞれの歯は5回の予約で治療され、そのつど根管内の細菌の存在が調べられた。それぞれの予約間には抗菌性貼薬剤は使用しなかった。0.5％次亜塩素酸ナトリウム溶液を使用すると、5回目の約束時には15根管中12根管で細菌が回収されなかった。この結果は、根管洗浄剤として生食水を使用したときの15根管中8根管と比較されるべきである。これらの結果は、0.5％次亜塩素酸ナトリウム溶液は根管洗浄剤として生食水よりも効果的であることを示唆していた。

（Oral Surg Oral Med Oral Pathol 1983；55（3）：307-312.）

The antibacterial effect of 0.5percent sodium hypochlorite solution as root canal irrigant was studied in fifteen single-rooted teeth. Each tooth was treated at five appointments, and the presence of bacteria in the root canal was studied on each occasion. No antibacterial intracanal dressings were used between the appointments. When 0.5percent hypochlorite was used no bacteria could be recovered from twelve of fifteen root canals at the fifth appointment. This should be compared with eight of fifteen root canals when saline solution was used as irrigant. These results suggest that 0.5percent sodium hypochlorite solution is more effective than saline solution as a root canal irrigant.

Endodontic irrigation

Biologic effects of dental materials. 3. Toxicity and antimicrobial effect of endodontic antiseptics *in vitro*.

歯科材料の生物学的効果
3．*in vitro* における根管消毒剤の毒性と抗菌効果

Spangberg L, Engström B, Langeland K.

　一般の歯内療法で用いられる種々の抗菌剤を、細胞毒性および殺菌効果という点において客観的測定法により評価した。すべての薬剤が、抗菌剤の細菌効果と比べて毒性が顕著であることがわかった。細胞毒性と殺菌効果、そして特定ニーズとの間のバランスに基づくと、適切な洗浄液や貼薬剤の使用が推奨される。

（Oral Surg Oral Med Oral Pathol 1973；36（6）：856-871.）

A number of commonly used endodontic antimicrobial agents were evaluated for cytotoxicity and bactericidal effect by an objective method. It was found that all medicaments were markedly toxic compared to their antimicrobial effect. On the basis of a balance between the cytotoxicity, the antimicrobial effect, and the specific needs, a recommendation for an adequate irrigation solution and a medicament for dressing is made.

A comparison of 2.0% chlorhexidine gluconate and 5.25% sodium hypochlorite as antimicrobial endodontic irrigants.

抗菌性根管洗浄剤としての2％グルコン酸クロルヘキシジンと5.25％次亜塩素酸ナトリウムの比較

Jeansonne MJ, White RR.

　根管洗浄剤としての次亜塩素酸ナトリウムは、毒性、臭い、および治療器具の変色という問題を有している。同等の抗菌効果をもち、より安全な洗浄剤が理想的である。したがって、われわれは、*in vitro* の根管系において、2.0％グルコン酸クロルヘキシジンの抗菌活性と5.25％次亜塩素酸ナトリウムの抗菌活性を比較した。歯髄病変のあるヒト新鮮抜去歯を、根管洗浄剤としてクロルヘキシジン、次亜塩素酸、または生食水を用いて根管形成した。細菌サンプルを、根管にアクセスした直後、根管形成洗浄後、そして嫌気的環境で24時間経過した後に、採取した。クロルヘキシジンあるいは次亜塩素酸ナトリウムでの根管洗浄は、生食水で洗浄した歯と比較して、洗浄後の細菌培養陽性数やコロニー形成単位（菌数）が有意に減少した。クロルヘキシジンで洗浄した歯から得られた陽性培養のうち、細菌培養陽性数やコロニー形成単位は次亜塩素酸で洗浄した歯と比較して少なかったが、その差には統計学的有意差は認められなかった。

（J Endod 1994；20（6）：276-278.）

Sodium hypochlorite, as an endodontic irrigant, poses problems including toxicity, odor, and discoloration of operatory items. An equally effective, but safer irrigant is desirable. Therefore, we compared the antimicrobial activity of 2.0% chlorhexidine gluconate with that of 5.25% sodium hypochlorite in an *in vitro* root canal system. Freshly extracted human teeth with pulpal pathosis were instrumented using chlorhexidine, sodium hypochlorite, or saline as irrigants. Microbiological samples were taken from the teeth immediately after accessing the canal, after instrumentation and irrigation, and after standing in an anaerobic atmosphere for 24h. Irrigation with chlorhexidine or sodium hypochlorite significantly reduced the numbers of postirrigant positive cultures and colony-forming units compared with saline-irrigated teeth. The number of postirrigant positive cultures and the number of colony-forming units in positive cultures obtained from chlorhexidine-treated teeth were lower than the numbers obtained from sodium hypochlorite-treated teeth, but the differences were not statistically significant.

Endodontic irrigation

Reduction of intracanal bacteria using nickel-titanium rotary instrumentation and various medications.

Ni-Ti 製ロータリーファイルの根管形成とさまざまな薬物を使用した根管内細菌の減少

Shuping GB, Orstavik D, Sigurdsson A, Trope M.

本研究の目的は、Ni-Ti 製ロータリーファイルと1.25％次亜塩素酸ナトリウムによる根管洗浄を併用したときの、細菌減少量を評価することである。本研究ではさらに、1週間以上の水酸化カルシウム貼薬による付加的抗菌効果についても検証した。慢性根尖性歯周炎のエックス線像と臨床症状を有する42歯の実験材料が集められた。根管は、術前、根管形成中、根管形成後、そして水酸化カルシウム貼薬後にサンプリングされ、採取したサンプルは37℃で7日間嫌気培養された。各サンプルの細菌は定量され、そしてその計算と比較には対数値を用いた。術前に採取したサンプルから感染根管であることがわかった。次亜塩素酸ナトリウムを洗浄剤として使用すると、滅菌生理食塩水と比較して、細菌の有意に著しい減少傾向が認められた（$P<0.05$）。次亜塩素酸ナトリウムを併用した根管形成後において、61.9％の根管が無菌であった。少なくとも1週間の水酸化カルシウム貼薬を行うと、92.5％の根管が無菌となった。この結果は次亜塩素酸ナトリウム洗浄のみの場合と比べ、有意に減少していた（$P<0.0001$）。本研究結果は、ロータリーファイルを併用した次亜塩素酸ナトリウムの根管洗浄は、歯内療法中に根管内細菌を減少させる重要なステップであることを示している。しかしながら、この手法では必ずしも根管を無菌にできなかった。より予見性をもって根管内を無菌化するという目標を達成するためには、本法に水酸化カルシウム貼薬を追加処置することが、望ましいと思われる。

（J Endod 2000；26（12）：751-755.）

The purpose of this study was to evaluate the extent of bacterial reduction with nickel-titanium rotary instrumentation and 1.25% NaOCl irrigation. Also, the additional antibacterial effect of calcium hydroxide for >1wk was tested. Forty-two subjects with radiographic and clinical signs of chronic apical periodontitis were recruited. The canals were sampled before treatment, during and after instrumentation, and after treatment with calcium hydroxide and the samples incubated anaerobically for 7days at 37degrees C. The bacteria from each sample were quantified and the log10 values were used for calculations and comparisons. The initial sample confirmed infection of the canals. There was a significantly greater pattern of reduction of bacteria when NaOCl was used as an irrigant, compared with sterile saline ($p<0.05$). After instrumentation with NaOCl irrigation, 61.9% of canals were rendered bacteria-free. The placement of calcium hydroxide for at least 1 wk rendered 92.5% of the canals bacteria free. This was a significant reduction, compared with NaOCl irrigation alone ($p<0.0001$). The results of this study indicate that NaOCl irrigation with rotary instrumentation is an important step in the reduction of canal bacteria during endodontic treatment. However this method could not consistently render canals bacteria-free. The addition of calcium hydroxide intracanal medication should be used to more predictably attain this goal.

エンドのための重要20キーワード

Sodium hypochlorite
次亜塩素酸ナトリウム

　機械的な清掃法に加えて、十分かつ適切な化学的清掃法（根管洗浄）を行うことは、歯内療法を成功へ導く重要な因子のひとつである。次亜塩素酸ナトリウムには組織溶解性（有機質溶解性）や消毒作用があり、現在においても、根管洗浄剤の主流である。本稿では、主に、次亜塩素酸ナトリウムの根管消毒効果に対して検索を行った論文を紹介する。

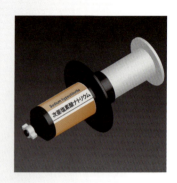

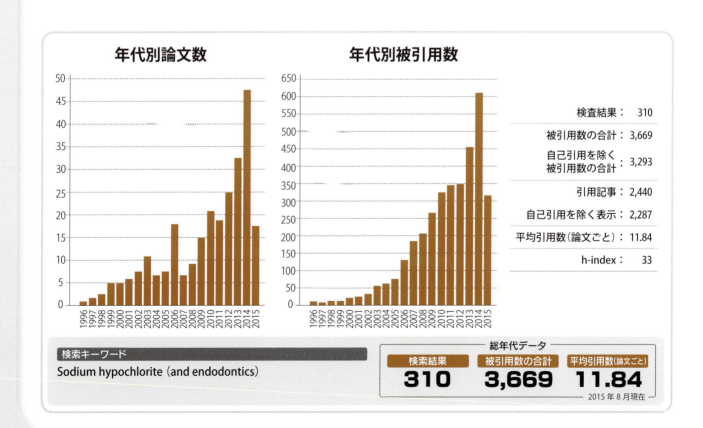

検索キーワード: Sodium hypochlorite (and endodontics)

検査結果: 310
被引用数の合計: 3,669
自己引用を除く被引用数の合計: 3,293
引用記事: 2,440
自己引用を除く表示: 2,287
平均引用数（論文ごと）: 11.84
h-index: 33

総年代データ
検索結果: 310
被引用数の合計: 3,669
平均引用数（論文ごと）: 11.84
2015年8月現在

'9 Sodium hypochlorite

トムソン・ロイターが選んだベスト**12**論文

	タイトル・和訳	2011年	2012年	2013年	2014年	合計引用数
引用数 **1**位	Torabinejad M, Handysides R, Khademi AA, Bakland LK. Clinical implications of the smear layer in endodontics : a review. Oral Surg Oral Med Oral Pathol Oral Radiol Endod 2002 ; 94(6) : 658-666. 歯内療法におけるスメヤー層の臨床的意味：総説論文 **本項に和訳あり**	15	8	12	17	160
引用数 **2**位	Gomes BP, Ferraz CC, Vianna ME, Berber VB, Teixeira FB, Souza-Filho FJ. In vitro antimicrobial activity of several concentrations of sodium hypochlorite and chlorhexidine gluconate in the elimination of Enterococcus faecalis. Int Endod J 2001 ; 34(6) : 424-428. Enterococcus faecalis 排除に関して次亜塩素酸とグルコン酸クロルヘキシジンをさまざまな濃度で使用した場合の in vitro における抗菌効果 **本項に和訳あり**	13	14	16	14	148
引用数 **3**位	Hülsmann M, Heckendorff M, Lennon A. Chelating agents in root canal treatment : mode of action and indications for their use. Int Endod J 2003 ; 36(12) : 810-830. 根管治療におけるキレート剤：作用機序と使用指針 **チャプター10に和訳あり**	14	16	19	14	143
引用数 **4**位	Safavi KE, Nichols FC. Effect of calcium hydroxide on bacterial lipopolysaccharide. J Endod 1993 ; 19(2) : 76-78. 細菌性リポ多糖（LPS）に対する水酸化カルシウムの効果	7	7	6	7	92
引用数 **5**位	Mohammadi Z, Abbott PV. The properties and applications of chlorhexidine in endodontics. Int Endod J 2009 ; 42(4) : 288-302. 歯内療法におけるクロルヘキシジンの特性および応用	12	19	25	15	91
引用数 **6**位	Clegg MS, Vertucci FJ, Walker C, Belanger M, Britto LR. The effect of exposure to irrigant solutions on apical dentin biofilms in vitro. J Endod 2006 ; 32(5) : 434-437. 根尖部バイオフィルムに対して根管洗浄剤を曝したときの in vitro における効果 **本項に和訳あり**	3	5	14	6	69

トムソン・ロイターが選んだベスト**12**論文

	タイトル・和訳	2011年	2012年	2013年	2014年	合計引用数
引用数 **7**位	Wu MK, Dummer PM, Wesselink PR. Consequences of and strategies to deal with residual post-treatment root canal infection. Int Endod J 2006；39（5）:343-356. 術後に残留感染を有する根管の今後と対処法	7	3	8	17	65
引用数 **8**位	Haapasalo M, Qian W, Portenier I, Waltimo T. Effects of dentin on the antimicrobial properties of endodontic medicaments. J Endod 2007；33（8）: 917-225. 歯内療法の薬剤の抗菌特性に対する象牙質の影響	6	6	14	7	64
引用数 **9**位	Radcliffe CE, Potouridou L, Qureshi R, Habahbeh N, Qualtrough A, Worthington H, Drucker DB. Antimicrobial activity of varying concentrations of sodium hypochlorite on the endodontic microorganisms *Actinomyces israelii*, *A. naeslundii*, *Candida albicans* and *Enterococcus faecalis*. Int Endod J 2004；37（7）: 438-446. 歯内療法に関係する細菌 *Actinomyces israeli*、*A-naeslundii*、*Candida albicans* および *Enterococcus faecalis* に対するさまざまな濃度の次亜塩素酸ナトリウムの抗菌活性　**本項に和訳あり**	6	5	4	11	64
引用数 **10**位	Guerisoli DM, Marchesan MA, Walmsley AD, Lumley PJ, Pecora JD. Evaluation of smear layer removal by EDTAC and sodium hypochlorite with ultrasonic agitation. Int Endod J 2002；35（5）: 418-421. EDTACと次亜塩素酸ナトリウムの超音波撹拌によるスメヤー層除去効果	6	10	9	8	63
引用数 **11**位	Violich DR, Chandler NP. The smear layer in endodontics — a review. Int Endod J 2010；43（1）: 2-15. 総説論文─歯内療法におけるスメヤー層	6	10	13	20	58
引用数 **12**位	Bergenholtz G, Spångberg L. Controversies in endodontics. Crit Rev Oral Biol Med 2004；15（2）: 99-114. 歯内療法における論点	3	1	7	3	54

Sodium hypochlorite

Clinical implications of the smear layer in endodontics: a review.

歯内療法におけるスメヤー層の臨床的意味：総説論文

Torabinejad M, Handysides R, Khademi AA, Bakland LK.

　根管壁表面を覆うスメヤー層が、根管形成により生じることは、何年もの間、認識されていた。この層は、象牙芽細胞の断片や壊死性残屑のような無機物質および有機物質を含んでいる。スメヤー層は、それ自体が感染しているかもしれず、また象牙細管内に存在する細菌を保護してしまうかもしれないのに、根管形成や根管充填の質におけるスメヤー層の影響に関して、いまだ統一的見解は得られていない。いろいろな手法がスメヤー層を除去するために用いられてきた。そして、スメヤー層があること、もしくはスメヤー層を取り去ることの意義に関し、多くの *in vitro* の研究から、相反する結果が報告されている。

（Oral Surg Oral Med Oral Pathol Oral Radiol Endod 2002；94（6）：658-666.）

It has been recognized for many years that root canal instrumentation produces a smear layer that covers the surfaces of prepared canal walls. This layer contains inorganic and organic substances such as fragments of odontoblastic processes and necrotic debris. There is a lack of agreement regarding the effect of the smear layer on the quality of instrumentation and obturation, but the smear layer itself may be infected and may protect the bacteria within the dentinal tubules. Various methods have been used to remove the smear layer. Conflicting results have been obtained from numerous *in vitro* studies regarding the significance of the presence or the removal of the smear layer.

In vitro antimicrobial activity of several concentrations of sodium hypochlorite and chlorhexidine gluconate in the elimination of *Enterococcus faecalis*.

Enterococcus faecalis 排除に関して次亜塩素酸とグルコン酸クロルヘキシジンをさまざまな濃度で使用した場合の *in vitro* における抗菌効果

Gomes BP, Ferraz CC, Vianna ME, Berber VB, Teixeira FB, Souza-Filho FJ.

目的：本研究の目的は、*in vitro* において、*E. faecalis* 排除に関する次亜塩素酸ナトリウム(0.5%、1%、2.5%、5.25%)および3つの濃度のグルコン酸クロルヘキシジンの両性状(ゲルと液状)の効果を評価することであった。　**方法**：24ウェル細胞培養用プレートを用いて液体希釈試験が実施され、各洗浄液が細菌細胞を死滅するのに要する時間が記録された。10%ヒツジ血液ブレインハートインフュージョン寒天培地において増殖させた *E. faecalis* の24時間純粋培養から単離したコロニーは、0.85%滅菌食塩液に懸濁された。細胞懸濁液はマクファーランド濁度標準液0.5番の濁度と一致するように分光光度的に調整された。それぞれの試験洗浄剤1 mLとコントロール群(滅菌生理食塩液)は、24ウェル細胞培養用プレート(Coming社)のウェルの底に置かれた。6ウェルを、各設定時間別および各洗浄剤濃度別に使用した。細胞懸濁液2 mLとそれぞれの洗浄剤を10秒間超音波混合した後、10秒、30秒、45秒、1分、3分、5分、10分、20分、30分、1時間および2時間、ウェルの洗浄剤上に置いた。各実験時間経過後、それぞれのウェルから1 mLを取りだし、洗浄剤の残留作用を防ぐために新たに調整した2 mLのBHI＋中和剤の入ったチューブに移した。すべてのチューブは37℃で7日間培養された。インキュベーション期間中に中程度の濁度を示したチューブを、増殖陽性が生じているチューブとした。データは Kruskal-Wallis 検定を用い有意水準0.05で統計学的に解析した。　**結果**：すべての洗浄剤は、*E. faecalis* の殺菌に効果的であった。しかし、殺菌効果が現れるまでの時間は異なっていた。テストしたすべての濃度(0.2%、1%、2%)で液状クロルヘキシジンと5.25%次亜塩素酸ナトリウムは、もっとも効果的な洗浄剤であった。しかし、0.2%液状クロルヘキシジンと2%ゲル状クロルヘキシジンが培養陰性となるのに要する時間は、それぞれ、たった30秒と1分であった。　**結論**：すべての洗浄剤は、抗菌活性を有していたが、*E. faecalis* を排除するために要する時間は検索した洗浄剤の濃度と性状に左右された。

(Int Endod J 2001 ; 34 (6) : 424-428.)

AIM: The aim of this study was to assess, *in vitro*, the effectiveness of several concentrations of NaOCl(0.5%, 1%, 2.5%, and 5.25%) and two forms of chlorhexidine gluconate (gel and liquid) in three concentrations (0.2%, 1% and 2%) in the elimination of *E. faecalis*.
METHODOLOGY: A broth dilution test using 24-well cell culture plates was performed and the time taken for the irrigants to kill bacterial cells was recorded. Isolated 24 h colonies of pure cultures of E. faecalis grown on 10% sheep blood plus Brain Heart Infusion (BHI) agar plates were suspended in sterile 0.85% NaCl solution. The cell suspension was adjusted spectrophotometrically to match the turbidity of a McFarland 0.5 scale. One mL of each tested substance was placed on the bottom of wells of 24-well cell culture plates (Corning, NY), including the control group (sterile saline). Six wells were used for each time period and irrigant concentration. Two mL of the bacterial suspension were ultrasonically mixed for 10 s with the irrigants and placed in contact with them for 10, 30, and 45 s ; 1, 3, 5, 10, 20, and 30 min ; and 1 and 2h. After each period of time, 1mL from each well was transferred to tubes containing 2mL of freshly prepared BHI+ neutralizers in order to prevent a residual action of the irrigants. All tubes were incubated at 37 degrees C for 7 days. The tubes considered to have positive growth were those which presented medium turbidity during the incubation period. Data were analysed statistically by the Kruskal-Wallis test. with the level of significance set at P<0.05.
RESULTS: All irrigants were effective in killing *E. faecalis*, but at different times. Chlorhexidine in the liquid form at all concentrations tested (0.2%, 1% and 2%) and NaOCl (5.25%) were the most effective irrigants. However, the time required by 0.2% chlorhexidine liquid and 2% chlorhexidine gel to promote negative cultures was only 30 s and 1min, respectively.
CONCLUSIONS: Even though all tested irrigants possessed antibacterial activity, the time required to eliminate *E. faecalis* depended on the concentration and type of irrigant used.

Sodium hypochlorite

The effect of exposure to irrigant solutions on apical dentin biofilms *in vitro*.

根尖部バイオフィルムに対して根管洗浄剤を曝したときの *in vitro* における効果

Clegg MS, Vertucci FJ, Walker C, Belanger M, Britto LR.

　本研究は異なる濃度の次亜塩素酸ナトリウム、2.0%クロルヘキシジン（Vista Dental Products）、BioPure MTAD（デンツプライ社）の洗浄効果を評価した。根管内容物を、慢性根尖性歯周炎と診断された患者10名から採取した。採取したサンプルを、複数菌よりなるバイオフィルムを生じさせるために根尖の片側切断面上で培養した。それぞれのバイオフィルムは、別々に、6.0%、3.0%および1.0%の次亜塩素酸ナトリウム、2.0%のクロルヘキシジン、1.0%の次亜塩素酸ナトリウムと BioPure MTAD の併用、および滅菌リン酸緩衝液（PBS）に浸漬した。6.0%および3.0%の次亜塩素酸ナトリウムがバイオフィルムを崩壊して除去できること、1.0%の次亜塩素酸ナトリウムと BioPure MTAD の併用は、バイオフィルムを崩壊できるが細菌を排除できないこと、そして2.0%のクロルヘキシジンはバイオフィルムを崩壊できないことが、走査型電子顕微鏡分析から示された。生菌は、6.0%の次亜塩素酸ナトリウム、2.0%のクロルヘキシジン、および1.0%の次亜塩素酸ナトリウムと BioPure MTAD の併用した根管洗浄液群に曝した試料からは、培養されなかった。これらの結果は、6.0%の次亜塩素酸ナトリウムが細菌を不活性化し、バイオフィルムを物理的に除去できる唯一の洗浄剤であることを示している。

（J Endod 2006；32（5）：434-437.）

This study assessed the effectiveness of different concentrations of sodium hypochlorite (NaOCl), 2% chlorhexidine (CHX)(Vista Dental Products, Racine, WI), and BioPure MTAD (Dentsply Endodontics-Tulsa Dental, Tulsa, OK). Intracanal contents were collected from 10 patients diagnosed with chronic apical periodontitis. The samples were cultured on hemisections of root apices to generate a polymicrobial biofilm. Each biofilm was separately immersed in 6% NaOCl, 3% NaOCl, 1% NaOCl, 2% CHX, 1% NaOCl followed by BioPure MTAD, and sterile phosphate buffered solution (PBS). SEM analysis showed 6% NaOCl and 3% NaOCl were capable of disrupting and removing the biofilm; 1% NaOCl and 1% NaOCl followed by MTAD were capable of disrupting the biofilm, but not eliminating bacteria; 2% CHX was not capable of disrupting the biofilm. Viable bacteria could not be cultured from specimens exposed to 6% NaOCl, 2% CHX, or 1% NaOCl followed by BioPure MTAD. These results indicate that 6% NaOCl was the only irrigant capable of both rendering bacteria nonviable and physically removing the biofilm.

Antimicrobial activity of varying concentrations of sodium hypochlorite on the endodontic microorganisms *Actinomyces israelii*, *A. naeslundii*, *Candida albicans* and *Enterococcus faecalis*.

歯内療法に関係する細菌 *Actinomyces israeli*、*A-naeslundii*、*Candida albicans* および *Enterococcus faecalis* に対するさまざまな濃度の次亜塩素酸ナトリウムの抗菌活性

Radcliffe CE, Potouridou L, Qureshi R, Habahbeh N, Qualtrough A, Worthington H, Drucker DB.

目的：難治性感染根管に関与する細菌の、根管洗浄剤次亜塩素酸ナトリウムに対する抵抗性を判定することを目的とした。

方法：2系統の *Actinomyces naeslundii*、*Candida albicans* および *Enterococcus faecalis* を、0.5％、1.0％、2.5％、および5.25％濃度（重量／容量に調整した次亜塩素酸ナトリウムに対して、対数増殖後期接種源として、試験した。実験に用いた接触時間は、0、10秒、20秒、30秒、60秒とした。*E. faecalis* の場合、追加実験として1分、2分、5分、10分、30分の接触時間を用いた。抗菌作用はチオ硫酸ナトリウム添加によって停止させた。まず、生菌を生菌数計測を用いてドロッププレート上生菌数計測を用いて測定した。次に、コロニー形成単位(cfu)の低い細菌を測定するためにポアプレート(pour-plates)を、そしてコロニー形成単位の大きい細菌を測定するために10^6倍の希釈を用いた。

結果：*A. naeslundii* および *C. albicans* に対する10秒以上の接触時間では、次亜塩素酸ナトリウムのすべての濃度で、測定限界より低いコロニー形成単位を示した。しかし、*E. faecalis* は次亜塩素酸ナトリウムに抵抗性がよりあることが示された。0.5％の次亜塩素酸ナトリウムを30分間作用させると、検査された *E. faecalis* 両系統においてコロニー形成単位はゼロに減少した。この結果は、1.0％の次亜塩素酸ナトリウム10分間、2.5％の次亜塩素酸ナトリウム5分間、および5.25％の次亜塩素酸ナトリウム2分間と比較して有意であった（$P<0.001$）。時間と菌数を従属変数 $\{\log(e)$（時間＋1）と $\log(e)$（菌数＋1）$\}$ と濃度を説明変数として回帰分析を行ったところ、時間と濃度の間に有意な相関が生じていた（$P<0.001$）。

結論：*E. faecalis* が観察された難治性歯内感染に関した症例報告は、このような次亜塩素酸ナトリウム高耐性の *E. faecalis* に、少なくとも何かしらの原因があるかもしれない。こうした報告は、*A. nacslundii* や *C. albicans* の症例ではないと思われる。

(Int Endod J 2004；37(7)：438-446.)

AIM: To determine the resistance of microorganisms associated with refractory endodontic infections to sodium hypochlorite used as a root canal irrigant.
METHODOLOGY: Two strains each of *Actinomyces naeslundii*, *Candida albicans* and *Enterococcus faecalis* were tested as late logarithmic phase inocula, against sodium hypochlorite adjusted to 0.5, 1.0, 2.5 and 5.25% w/v. Contact times used were 0, 10, 20, 30, 60 and 120 s. In the case of *E. faecalis*, additional experiments used contact times of 1.0, 2.0, 5.0, 10.0 and 30.0 min. Anti-microbial action was halted by sodium thiosulphate addition. Survivors were measured primarily using viable counts on drop plates. Additionally, pour plates were used to count low colony-forming units (cfu) and dilutions to 10 (-6) were used to count high cfu.
RESULTS: All concentrations of NaOCl lowered cfu below the limit of detection after 10 s in the case of *A. naeslundii* and *C.albicans*. However, *E. faecalis* proved to be more resistant to NaOCl. Using 0.5% NaOCl for 30 min reduced cfu to zero for both strains tested. his compares with 10 min for 1.0%, 5 min for 2.5% and 2 min for 5.25%(P<0.001). Regression analysis for the dependent variable log (e) (count +1) with log (e) (time+1) and concentration as explanatory variables gave rise to a significant interaction between time and concentration (P<0.001).
CONCLUSION: The published association of *E. faecalis* with refractory endodontic infection may result, at least partially, from high resistance of this species to NaOCl. This does not appear to be the case with *A.naeslundii* or *C.albicans*.

エンドのための重要20キーワード

10 EDTA

EDTA

根管洗浄の主たる目的は、根管内のスメヤー層や象牙質削片の除去、壊死組織の除去、および細菌の除去である。次亜塩素酸ナトリウムには組織溶解性があり、それなりの清掃効果は有している。しかしスメヤー層に対する次亜塩素酸ナトリウムの除去効果は、必ずしも優れていない。そのため、次亜塩素酸ナトリウム溶液とキレート剤EDTAを併用し、スメヤー層の除去を行うことが根管洗浄の趨勢となりつつある。本稿では、スメヤー層の除去に対するEDTAの効果を検索した論文を、主に紹介する。

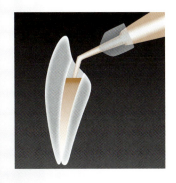

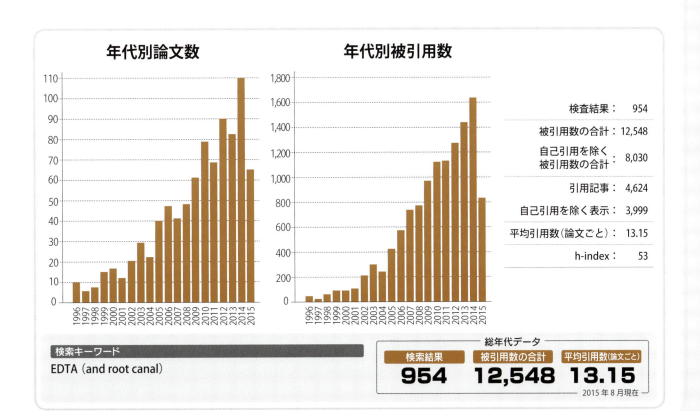

年代別論文数

年代別被引用数

検査結果：	954
被引用数の合計：	12,548
自己引用を除く被引用数の合計：	8,030
引用記事：	4,624
自己引用を除く表示：	3,999
平均引用数（論文ごと）：	13.15
h-index：	53

検索キーワード
EDTA（and root canal）

総年代データ

検索結果	被引用数の合計	平均引用数（論文ごと）
954	12,548	13.15

2015年8月現在

トムソン・ロイターが選んだベスト12論文

引用数	タイトル・和訳	2011年	2012年	2013年	2014年	合計引用数
1位	Bystrom A, Sundqvist G. The antibacterial action of sodium hypochlorite and EDTA in 60 cases of endodontic therapy. Int Endod J 1985；18(1)：35-40. 歯内治療した60症例における次亜塩素酸ナトリウムとEDTAの抗菌作用 **本項に和訳あり**	18	21	18	12	314
2位	Haapasalo M, Orstavik D. *In vitro* infection and disinfection of dentinal tubules. J Dent Res 1987；66(8)：1375-1379. *In vitro*における象牙細管の感染と消毒 **チャプター11に和訳あり**	12	18	15	27	299
3位	Nair PN, Henry S, Cano V, Vera J. Microbial status of apical root canal system of human mandibular first molars with primary apical periodontitis after"one-visit"endodontic treatment. Oral Surg Oral Med Oral Pathol Oral Radiol Endod 2005；99(2)：231-252. 1回治療法を用いた歯内療法後の初発根尖病変を有するヒト下顎第一大臼歯根尖部根管系の細菌学的状態 **チャプター8に和訳あり**	31	27	27	27	256
4位	Orstavik D, Haapasalo M. Disinfection by endodontic irrigants and dressings of experimentally infected dentinal tubules. Endod Dent Traumatol 1990；6(4)：142-149. 実験的感染象牙細管の歯内療法用洗浄剤と貼薬剤による消毒	4	5	13	6	230
5位	Torabinejad M, Khademi AA, Babagoli J, Cho Y, Johnson WB, Bozhilov K, Kim J, Shabahang S. A new solution for the removal of the smear layer. J Endod 2003；29(3)：170-175. スメヤー層除去に対する新溶液	16	19	19	9	177
6位	Calt S, Serper A. Time-dependent effects of EDTA on dentin structures. J Endod 2002；28(1)：17-19. 象牙質構造に及ぼすEDTAの時間依存性作用 **本項に和訳あり**	14	13	18	10	149

トムソン・ロイターが選んだベスト12論文

	タイトル・和訳	2011年	2012年	2013年	2014年	合計引用数
引用数 7位	Hülsmann M, Heckendorff M, Lennon A. Chelating agents in root canal treatment: mode of action and indications for their use. Int Endod J 2003; 36(12): 810-830. 根管治療におけるキレート剤：作用機序と使用指針 **本項に和訳あり**	14	16	19	14	143
引用数 8位	Sen BH, Wesselink PR, Türkün M. The smear layer: a phenomenon in root canal therapy. Int Endod J 1995; 28(3): 141-148. スメヤー層：根管治療における事象	5	6	7	7	126
引用数 9位	Peciuliene V, Balciuniene I, Eriksen HM, Haapasalo M. Isolation of *Enterococcus faecalis* in previously root-filled canals in a Lithuanian population. J Endod 2000; 26(10): 593-595. リトアニア人の既充填根管における *Enterococcus faecalis* の分離	8	15	10	3	115
引用数 10位	Takeda FH, Harashima T, Kimura Y, Matsumoto K. A comparative study of the removal of smear layer by three endodontic irrigants and two types of laser. Int Endod J 1999; 32(1): 32-39. 3種の根管洗浄剤と2タイプのレーザーによるスメヤー層除去に関する比較試験 **本項に和訳あり**	5	7	6	6	101
引用数 11位	Tay FR, Loushine RJ, Weller RN, Kimbrough WF, Pashley DH, Mak YF, Lai CN, Raina R, Williams MC. Ultrastructural evaluation of the apical seal in roots filled with a polycaprolactone-based root canal filling material. J Endod 2005; 31(7): 514-519. ポリカプロラクトン根管充填材を用いて根管充填したときの根尖部封鎖性の超微形態学的評価	6	5	4	6	98
引用数 12位	Torabinejad M, Cho Y, Khademi AA, Bakland LK, Shabahang S. The effect of various concentrations of sodium hypochlorite on the ability of MTAD to remove the smear layer. J Endod 2003; 29(4): 233-239. MTADのスメヤー層除去能に対する種々の次亜塩素酸ナトリウムの影響	10	9	8	5	96

The antibacterial action of sodium hypochlorite and EDTA in 60 cases of endodontic therapy.

歯内治療した60症例における次亜塩素酸ナトリウムとEDTAの抗菌作用

Bystrom A, Sundqvist G.

　0.5％と5％の次亜塩素酸ナトリウムで感染根管を洗浄した場合の抗菌効果が、本研究において臨床的に評価された。結果は、どちらの濃度の次亜塩素酸ナトリウム液においても抗菌効果には差がないことを示していた。EDTAと5％次亜塩素酸ナトリウムの両者を使うと、次亜塩素酸ナトリウムのみ使用したときより、さらに効果的であった。根管形成や根管洗浄後に生き残った細菌は、根管貼薬をしない場合、急速に増殖してしまうことが、重要な所見として挙げられた。

(Int Endod J 1985；18(1)：35-40.)

In this study the antibacterial effect of irrigating infected root canals with 0.5 and 5 percent sodium hypochlorite solutions was evaluated clinically. The results indicated that there was no difference between the antibacterial effect of these two solutions. The combined use of EDTA and S per cent sodium hypochlorite solution was more efficient than the use of sodium hypochlorite solutions alone. An important observation was that bacteria surviving instrumentation and irrigation rapidly increased in number in the period between appointments when no intracanal medicament was used.

Time-dependent effects of EDTA on dentin structures.

象牙質構造に及ぼす EDTA の時間依存性作用

Calt S, Serper A.

　本研究の目的は、EDTA 適用 1 分および10分後のスメヤー層の除去と象牙質構造に及ぼす EDTA の効果を評価することであった。6 本の単根抜去歯は60号で根管形成された。それぞれの根の根尖側 1 / 3 と歯冠側 1 / 3 は根中央部を残して取り除かれた。それから同じ大きさの 2 つの切片に歯軸方向で切断された。同じ歯根から 2 等分したそれぞれの切片は、10mL の17% EDTA を用いて、それぞれ 1 分および10分間洗浄された。その後、すべての試料は、走査型電子顕微鏡評価に供された。結果は、1 分間の EDTA 洗浄がスメヤー層の除去に効果的であることを示していた。しかし、10分間 EDTA を適用すると細管周囲、そして細管内の象牙質の過剰な浸食が生じていた。以上のことから、根管治療では 1 分以上この洗浄法を行うべきでないことが示唆された。

（J Endod 2002；28（1）：17-19.）

The purpose of this study was to evaluate the effects of EDTA on smear layer removal and on the structure of dentin, after 1 and 10 min of application. Six extracted single-rooted teeth were instrumented to #60. Apical and coronal thirds of each root were removed, leaving a 5mm middle third that was then cut longitudinally into two equal segments. Using 10mL of 17% EDTA solution, halves belonging to the same root were irrigated for 1 and 10 min, respectively. All specimens were subjected to irrigation with 10mL of 5% NaOCl. Then all the specimens were prepared for SEM evaluation. The results showed that 1 min EDTA irrigation is effective in removing the smear layer. However a 10-min application of EDTA caused excessive peritubular and intertubular dentinal erosion. Therefore we suggest that this procedure should not be prolonged >1 min during endodontic treatment.

Chelating agents in root canal treatment: mode of action and indications for their use.

根管治療のおけるキレート剤：作用機序と使用指針

Hülsmann M, Heckendorff M, Lennon A.

　キレート剤は、1957年 Nygaard-Östby によって、狭窄や石灰化した根管の根管形成の補助剤として歯内療法分野に導入された。エチレンジアミン四酢酸溶液（EDTA）は、象牙質透過性を増すだけでなく、根管象牙質を化学的に軟化し、そしてスメヤー層を溶解すると考えられている。根管象牙質を軟化することを目的とするEDTA製剤の有効性については討論されてきたが、キレート剤を用いた根管形成は近年再び人気を取り戻している。ほとんどすべての Ni-Ti 製ファイル製造元は、回転切削による根管形成中は潤滑剤としてキレート剤の使用を推奨している。加えて、多くの教科書で、スメヤー層除去を目的とする15%〜17% EDTA 溶液を用いた根管の最終洗浄が推奨されている。本論文は、キレート剤に関する論文を概説し、EDTA 製剤の化学的および薬理学的特性の概要を示し、そして EDTA の臨床使用指針を策定する。

(Int Endod J 2003；36(12)：810-830.)

Chelating agents were introduced into endodontics as an aid for the preparation of narrow and calcified root canals in 1957 by Nygaard-Østby. A liquid solution of ethylenediaminetetraacetic acid (EDTA) was thought to chemically soften the root canal dentine and dissolve the smear layer, as well as to increase dentine permeability. Although the efficacy of EDTA preparations in softening root dentine has been debated, chelator preparations have regained popularity recently. Almost all manufacturers of nickel-titanium instruments recommend their use as a lubricant during rotary root canal preparation. Additionally, a final irrigation of the root canal with 15-17% EDTA solutions to dissolve the smear layer is recommended in many textbooks. This paper reviews the relevant literature on chelating agents, presents an overview of the chemical and pharmacological properties of EDTA preparations and makes recommendations for their clinical use.

A comparative study of the removal of smear layer by three endodontic irrigants and two types of laser.

3種の根管洗浄剤と2タイプのレーザーによるスメヤー層除去に関する比較試験

Takeda FH, Harashima T, Kimura Y, Matsumoto K.

目的：根中央部と根尖部根管における、手用ファイルの根管形成により生じたスメヤー層に対する3種の根管洗浄剤および2種のレーザーの効果が *in vitro* において評価された。　**方法**：単根で狭い根尖口を有するヒト永久歯の下顎小臼歯抜去歯60歯は、それぞれの実験群が12歯となるように、5つの群に無作為に分類された。ステップバック法を用いてMAF60号で根管清掃・形成を行う際、それぞれのファイルサイズごとに根管を3mLの5.25% NaOClと3% H_2O_2 を用いて交互洗浄した。実験群1は、17% EDTAによる最終洗浄を行ったコントロールの試料とした。実験群2の歯はリン酸により、実験群3はクエン酸により最終洗浄を行った。実験群4の試料の根管は炭酸ガス（CO_2）レーザーで、実験群5の試料はEr:YAGレーザーを用いて洗浄された。歯は歯軸方向に割断された後、走査型電子顕微鏡検査に供された。
結果：コントロールの試料（実験群1）は根中央部根管において象牙細管の開口したきれいな根管壁を示したが、根尖部根管においては、いくつかの標本で厚いスメヤー層が観察された。6％リン酸（実験群2）あるいは6％クエン酸（実験群3）で最終洗浄された試料は、17% EDTAより根中央部根管において非常にきれいな根管面を示したが、根尖部において、とくに根尖開口部の象牙細管では、スメヤー層は完全には取り除かれていなかった。炭酸ガス（CO_2）レーザー（実験群4）で洗浄された試料は、根中央部と根尖部根管の両方で、スメヤー層のない、焦げて溶けて再結晶化し、かつ光滑なきれいな根管壁を呈していた。Er:YAGレーザー（実験群5）で洗浄された試料の根管壁は、根中央部と根尖部根管において、象牙細管は開口しており、スメヤー層のないことが明らかであった。統計学的解析は、実験群1と実験群2の間において、そして実験群1と実験群3の間において、統計学的な有意差は認められなかった。しかしながら、実験群1と実験群4の間と、実験群1と実験群5の間において、根中央部と根尖部根管における洗浄度に、統計学的な有意差が認められた（$P<0.01$）。　**結論**：17% EDTA、6％リン酸、および6％クエン酸は根管系からすべてのスメヤー層を取り除くことはできなかった。さらに、これらの酸性溶液は、象牙細管開口部の周囲の内側部象牙質を脱灰し、そしてその結果、象牙細管開口部が大きくなっていた。炭酸ガス（CO_2）レーザーは形成後の根管壁のスメヤー層を取り除き、溶解するのに有効であり、そしてEr:YAGレーザーは、根管壁からスメヤー層を除去するのにもっとも効果的であった。

(Int Endod J 1999；32（1）：32-39.)

AIM: The effects of three endodontic irrigants and two types of laser on a smear layer created by hand instrumentation were evaluated in vitro in the middle and apical thirds of root canals.
METHODOLOGY: Sixty human mature extracted mandibular premolar teeth with a single root canal and a closed apex were distributed randomly into five groups of 12 teeth each. Whilst cleaning and shaping up to a size 60 master apical file with a step-back technique, the root canals were irrigated with 3mL of 5.25% NaOCl and 3% H_2O_2, alternately, between each file size. Group1 (G1) were control specimens that were irrigated with a final flush of 17% EDTA. The teeth in group2 (G2) were irrigated with a final flush of 6% phosphoric acid, and group3 (G3) with 6% citric acid. In the specimens of group4 (G4) the root canals were irradiated with a carbon dioxide (CO_2) laser, and specimens of group5 (G5) were irradiated using an Er:YAG laser. The teeth were split longitudinally and prepared for examination by scanning electron microscopy.
RESULT: Control specimens (G1) showed clean root-canal walls with open dentinal tubules in the middle one-third, but in some specimens thick smear layer was observed in the apical one-third. Specimens irrigated with a final flush of 6% phosphoric acid (G2) or 6% citric acid (G3) were cleaner than with 17% EDTA, showing very clean root canal surfaces in the middle one-third but in the apical one-third the smear layer was not completely removed, especially at the openings of the dentinal tubules. The specimens irradiated with the CO_2 laser (G4) showed clean root-canal walls with the smear layer absent, charred, melted, recrystallized and glazed in both middle and apical thirds. The root-canal walls of the specimens irradiated with the Er:YAG laser (G5) revealed an absent smear layer with open dentinal tubules in the middle and apical thirds. Statistical analysis showed no significant difference in the cleanliness of root-canal wall between G1 and G2, and G1 and G3. However, there were statistically significant differences ($P<0.01$) between G1 and G4, and G1 and G5 in the cleanliness of the middle and apical one-thirds of the root canals.
CONCLUSIONS: Irrigation with 17% EDTA, 6% phosphoric acid and 6% citric acid did not remove all the smear layer from the root-canal system. In addition, these acidic solutions demineralized the interbular dentine around tabular openings, which became enlarged. The CO_2 laser was useful in removing and melting the smear layer on the instrumented root-canal walls and the Er:YAG laser was the most effective in removing the smear layer from the root-canal wall.

エンドのための重要20キーワード

11 Calcium hydroxide
水酸化カルシウム

　従前の歯内療法においては、ホルムクレゾール(FC)などの強力な消毒・殺菌効果を有する根管貼薬剤が主流であったが、発がん性、組織刺激性などの観点から、次第に使用されなくなりつつある。そこで登場した水酸化カルシウムは、1985年頃普及し始めた貼薬剤で、現在、もっとも普及している根管貼薬剤のひとつである。高アルカリ性であるため、殺菌効果が期待できるとともに、根尖部における炎症の治癒に効果がある。壊死組織の溶解、滲出液の抑制、炎症の消炎、および硬組織の誘導作用などの効果が期待できるといわれている。本項においては、水酸化カルシウムを貼薬剤として用いたときの効果を検索した論文を、主に紹介する。

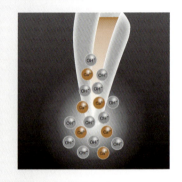

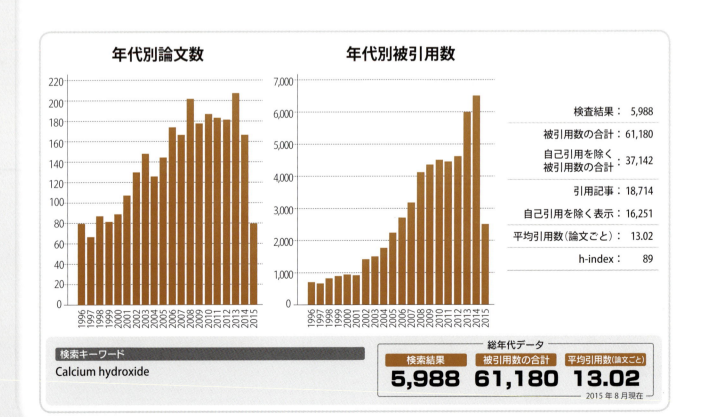

検索キーワード: Calcium hydroxide

検査結果: 5,988
被引用数の合計: 61,180
自己引用を除く被引用数の合計: 37,142
引用記事: 18,714
自己引用を除く表示: 16,251
平均引用数(論文ごと): 13.02
h-index: 89

総年代データ
検索結果: 5,988　被引用数の合計: 61,180　平均引用数(論文ごと): 13.02

2015年8月現在

⑪ Calcium hydroxide

トムソン・ロイターが選んだベスト**12**論文

	タイトル・和訳	2011年	2012年	2013年	2014年	合計引用数
引用数 **1位**	Sundqvist G, Figdor D, Persson S, Sjögren U. Microbiologic analysis of teeth with failed endodontic treatment and the outcome of conservative re-treatment. Oral Surg Oral Med Oral Pathol Oral Radiol Endod 1998；85（1）：86-93. 歯内療法を失敗した歯の細菌学的解析と再保存治療の治療成績 **チャプター15に和訳あり**	31	38	39	36	547
引用数 **2位**	Bystrom A, Claesson R, Sundqvist G. The antibacterial effect of camphorated paramonochlorophenol, camphorated phenol and calcium hydroxide in the treatment of infected root canals. Endod Dent Traumatol 1985；1（5）：170-175. 感染根管治療におけるCMCP、フェノールカンフル、および水酸化カルシウムの抗菌効果 **本項に和訳あり**	13	15	20	9	381
引用数 **3位**	Zehnder M. Root canal irrigants. J Endod 2006；32（5）：389-398. 根管洗浄剤	44	38	61	51	347
引用数 **4位**	Haapasalo M, Orstavik D. *In vitro* infection and disinfection of dentinal tubules. J Dent Res 1987；66（8）：1375-1379. *In vitro* における象牙細管の感染と消毒 **本項に和訳あり**	12	18	15	27	299
引用数 **5位**	Sjögren U, Figdor D, Spångberg L, Sundqvist G. The antimicrobial effect of calcium hydroxide as a short-term intracanal dressing. Int Endod J 1991；24（3）：119-125. 短期間根管貼薬したときの水酸化カルシウムの抗菌効果 **本項に和訳あり**	17	14	15	12	269
引用数 **6位**	Nair PN, Henry S, Cano V, Vera J. Microbial status of apical root canal system of human mandibular first molars with primary apical periodontitis after"one-visit"endodontic treatment. Oral Surg Oral Med Oral Pathol Oral Radiol Endod 2005；99（2）：231-252. １回治療法を用いた歯内療法後の初発根尖病変を有するヒト下顎第一大臼歯根尖部根管系の細菌学的状態 **チャプター８に和訳あり**	31	27	27	27	256

エンドのための重要20キーワード（関連性の高い論文和訳）

トムソン・ロイターが選んだベスト12論文

	タイトル・和訳	2011年	2012年	2013年	2014年	合計引用数
引用数 7位	Schröder U. Effects of calcium hydroxide-containing pulp-capping agents on pulp cell migration, proliferation, and differentiation. J Dent Res 1985；64：541-548. 歯髄細胞の遊走、増殖、および分化に対する水酸化カルシウム含有覆髄剤の効果	8	16	13	15	242
引用数 8位	Tronstad L, Andreasen JO, Hasselgren G, Kristerson L, Riis I. pH changes in dental tissues after root canal filling with calcium hydroxide. J Endod 1981；7（1）：17-21. 水酸化カルシウムで根管充填した後の歯科組織のpH変化	15	11	10	7	229
引用数 9位	Banchs F, Trope M. Revascularization of immature permanent teeth with apical periodontitis：new treatment protocol？ J Endod 2004；30（4）：196-200. 根尖性歯周炎をともなう幼若永久歯のリバスクラリセーション：新しい治療のプロトコール？ **チャプター18に和訳あり**	23	23	43	44	206
引用数 10位	Tziafas D, Smith AJ, Lesot H. Designing new treatment strategies in vital pulp therapy. J Dent 2000；28（2）：77-92. 生活歯髄療法における新しい治療の設計戦略	17	15	11	10	201
引用数 11位	Andreasen JO, Farik B, Munksgaard EC. Long-term calcium hydroxide as a root canal dressing may increase risk of root fracture. Dent Traumatol 2002；18（3）：134-137. 根管貼薬剤としての水酸化カルシウム長期貼薬は歯根破折の危険性を増す可能性がある **本項に和訳あり**	26	24	30	35	197
引用数 12位	Siqueira JF Jr, Lopes HP. Mechanisms of antimicrobial activity of calcium hydroxide：a critical review. Int Endod J 1999；32（5）：361-369. 水酸化カルシウムの抗菌活性のメカニズム：批評的総説	16	12	20	22	191

Calcium hydroxide

The antibacterial effect of camphorated paramonochlorophenol, camphorated phenol and calcium hydroxide in the treatment of infected root canals.

感染根管治療におけるCMCP、フェノールカンフル、および水酸化カルシウムの抗菌効果

Bystrom A, Claesson R, Sundqvist G.

　根尖病変を有する65歯の単根歯の根管を治療したときの、根管貼薬剤として用いた水酸化カルシウム、フェノールカンフル、およびCMCP（camphorated paramonochlorophenol）の殺菌効果を臨床的に評価した。根管内の少数の嫌気性菌も検出可能な細菌学的技法を用いた。水酸化カルシウムペースト（Calasept）根管貼薬剤を用いた治療後において、細菌は治療した35根管のうちの1根管から回収された。根管貼薬剤としてフェノールカンフル、あるいはCMCPを使用した後は、細菌は治療した30根管のうちの10根管から回収された。治療に抵抗性のある特異な細菌は明らかにならなかった。その結果は、感染根管治療は根管貼薬剤として水酸化カルシウムペーストを使用すると2回の治療で終了できることを示していた。

（Endod Dent Traumatol 1985；1（5）：170-175.）

The bactericidal efficacy of calcium hydroxide, camphorated phenol and camphorated paramonochlorophenol as intracanal dressings was evaluated clinically when the root canals of 65 single-rooted teeth with periapical lesions were treated. A bacteriological technique that could detect even small numbers of anaerobic bacteria in the canals was used. After treatment, including intracanal dressing with calcium hydroxide paste (Calasept), bacteria were recovered from one of 35 treated root canals. After use of camphorated phenol or camphorated paramonochlorophenol as the dressing. bacteria were recovered from 10 of 30 treated root canals. The isolated bacteria were predominantly Gram-positive and anaerobic. There was no indication that specific bacteria were resistant to the treatment. The results indicate that the endodontic treatment of infected root canals can be completed in two appointments when calcium hydroxide paste is used as an intracanal dressing.

In vitro infection and disinfection of dentinal tubules.

In vitro における象牙細管の感染と消毒

Haapasalo M, Orstavik D.

　根管における象牙細管の感染の*in vitro*実験模型が開発された。直径6mm、根管径2.3mm、高さ4mmの筒状の象牙質試料は、新鮮抜去ウシ切歯より作成された。セメント質は、すべての象牙質ブロックから取り除かれた。酵母エキスグルコースブイヨン中の*Enterococcus faecalis* ATCC 29212を感染させる前に、17%EDTAと5.25%次亜塩素酸ナトリウムで4分間処理し、細管を開口した。細菌は急速に細管へ浸潤した。3週間後、重度の感染は根管腔から400μmの位置でも観察され、いくつかのブロックでは感染の最前部は1,000μmに達していた。CMCP（Camphorated paramonochlorophenol）および水酸化カルシウム製剤（Calasept）の*E. faecalis*に感染した象牙質に対するそれぞれの薬剤の消毒効果を検査した。液状のCMCPはすばやく完全に象牙細管を消毒した。一方、ガス状のCMCPは液状のCMCPほど急速に象牙細管を消毒しなかった。Calaseptは、細管内の*E. faecalis*を、細管表層でさえ排除することはできなかった。本研究で細菌の採取に用いた手法は、根中央から外周へ100μmまでの象牙質を連続的に取り除くことを可能にした。コントロールの試料は、一律に感染しており、バー標本状の細菌の増殖はバーの表面から最大500μmに達していた。本実験の模型は、きわめて高感度に分析が可能であったことから、*in vitro*における根管貼薬剤の検査に適していると思われる。

（J Dent Res 1987；66（8）：1375-1379.）

An *in vitro* model for dentinal tubule infection of root canals was developed. Cylindrical dentin specimens, 4mm high with a diameter of 6mm and a canal 2.3mm wide, were prepared from freshly extracted bovine incisors. The cementum was removed from all dentin blocks. The tubules were opened by four-minute treatments with 17% EDTA and 5.25% NaOCl before being infected with *Enterococcus faecalis* ATCC 29212 in yeast extract-glucose broth. Bacteria rapidly invaded the tubules. After three weeks of incubation, a heavy infection was found 400 micron from the canal lumen, and the front of the infection reached 1000 micron in some blocks. Camphorated paramonochlorophenol (CMCP) and a calcium hydroxide compound, Calasept, were tested for their disinfecting efficacy toward *E. faecalis*-infected dentin. Liquid CMCP rapidly and completely disinfected the dentinal tubules, whereas CMCP in gaseous form disinfected tubules less rapidly. Calasept failed to eliminate, even superficially, *E. faecalis* in the tubules. The method used in bacteriological sampling allowed for sequential removal of 100-micron-thick zones of dentin from the central canal toward the periphery. Control specimens were uniformly infected and yielded growth in bur samples up to some 500 microns from the surface. The model proved quite sensitive and seems suitable for *in vitro* testing of root canal medicaments.

Calcium hydroxide

The antimicrobial effect of calcium hydroxide as a short-term intracanal dressing.

短期間根管貼薬したときの水酸化カルシウムの抗菌効果

Sjögren U, Figdor D, Spångberg L, Sundqvist G.

短期間、根管貼薬したときの水酸化カルシウムの抗菌効果を、根尖病巣を有する歯の根管内に10分間または7日間貼薬することより臨床的に評価した。7日間の貼薬は、根管の機械的清掃で生き残った細菌を効果的に除去した。一方、10分間の貼薬では、細菌の除去効果がないという結果が示された。

(Int Endod J 1991;24(3):119-125.)

The antibacterial effect of calcium hydroxide as a short-term intracanal dressing was clinically evaluated by applying the medicament for 10 minutes or 7days in root canals of teeth with periapical lesions. The results showed that the 7-day dressing efficiently eliminated bacteria which survived biomechanical instrumentation of the canal, while the 10-minute application was ineffective.

Long-term calcium hydroxide as a root canal dressing may increase risk of root fracture.

根管貼薬剤としての水酸化カルシウム長期貼薬は歯根破折の危険性を増す可能性がある

Andreasen JO, Farik B, Munksgaard EC.

　幼若歯は水酸化カルシウムが貼薬され、ガッタパーチャで根管充填されると脆くなることが1992年にCvekにより提唱された。本研究の目的は、水酸化カルシウムと接した象牙質は、ある一定期間経過後に破折強度の減少を示すという仮説を調べることであった。ヒツジの下顎幼若切歯は抜歯され、そして2つの実験群に分類された。実験群1として、歯髄は根尖口で抜髄した。その後、根管を水酸化カルシウムで充填し、IRM(R)セメントで封鎖した後、それらの歯は、室温で0.5、1、2、3、6、9、あるいは12か月生理食塩液中に保管された。実験群2として、歯髄を抜髄したあと、生理食塩液で満たし、IRM(R)セメントで封鎖した。それらの歯は2か月間生理食塩液中に保管された。コントロールとして用いた健全歯は抜歯後、すぐに試験された。すべての歯は、指定の観察期間経過後にインストロン型試験機で破折強度が検査された。その試験結果は、保管時間の増加とともに実験群1（水酸化カルシウム貼薬群）の破折強度が明らかに減少することを示していた。その試験結果は、水酸化カルシウムが充填された幼若歯の破折強度は、その水酸化カルシウムによる充填のためにおよそ1年間で半分になるであろうことを示していた。この所見は、しばしば症例報告として見受けられる長期間水酸化カルシウムで充填された幼若歯の破折について説明してくれるかもしれない。

（Dent Traumatol 2002；18（3）：134-137.）

It has been proposed (Cvek 1992) that immature teeth are weakened by filling of the root canals with calcium hydroxide dressing and gutta-percha. The aim of the present study was to test the hypothesis that dentin in contact with calcium hydroxide would show a reduction in fracture strength after a certain period of time. Immature mandibular incisors from sheep were extracted and divided into two experimental groups. Group1:the pulps were extirpated via the apical foramen. The root canals were then filled with calcium hydroxide (Calasept) and sealed with IRM (R) cement, and the teeth were then stored in saline at room temperature for 0.5, 1, 2, 3, 6, 9, or 12 months. Group2: the pulps were extirpated and the root canals were filled with saline and sealed with IRM (R) cement. The teeth were then stored in saline for 2 months. Intact teeth served as controls and were tested immediately after extraction. All teeth were tested for fracture strength in an Instron testing machine at the indicated observation periods. The results showed a markedly decrease in fracture strength with increasing storage time for group1 (calcium hydroxide dressing). The results indicate that the fracture strength of calcium hydroxide-filled immature teeth will be halved in about a year due to the root filling. The finding may explain the frequent reported fractures of immature teeth filled with calcium hydroxide for extended periods.

エンドのための重要20キーワード

12 Root canal condensation
根管充填

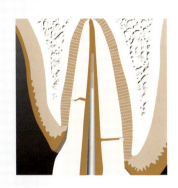

歯内療法は、機械的清掃法（根管形成）や化学的清掃法（根管洗浄）を用いて、根管内をできる限りきれいにした後、根管充填を用いて、根管内に新たな感染が生じないようにする一連の治療である。根管充填では、とくに感染根管治療において、化学的機械的根管形成（chemomechanical root canal preparation）では除去しきれなかった細菌などの感染源を封じ込める効果も期待される。そのため、以前から、より緊密で封鎖性の優れた根管充填材や根管充填法を検索したさまざまな研究が報告されている。

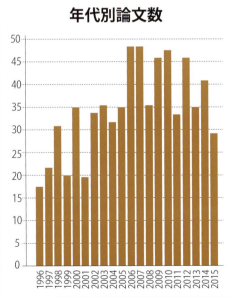

年代別論文数

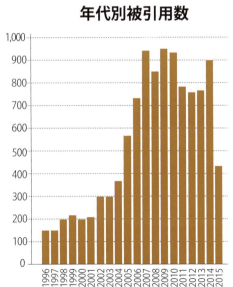

年代別被引用数

検査結果：	955
被引用数の合計：	11,422
自己引用を除く被引用数の合計：	8,157
引用記事：	4,074
自己引用を除く表示：	3,563
平均引用数（論文ごと）：	11.96
h-index：	46

検索キーワード
Root canal condensation

総年代データ
検索結果	被引用数の合計	平均引用数（論文ごと）
955	11,422	11.96

2015年8月現在

トムソン・ロイターが選んだベスト12論文

	タイトル・和訳	2011年	2012年	2013年	2014年	合計引用数
引用数 1位	Shipper G, Ørstavik D, Teixeira FB, Trope M. An evaluation of microbial leakage in roots filled with a thermoplastic synthetic polymer-based root canal filling material (Resilon). J Endod 2004;30(5):342-347. 熱可塑性合成ポリマー製根管充填材(レジロン)で根管充填された歯の微小漏洩の評価 **本項に和訳あり**	20	19	15	11	273
引用数 2位	Torabinejad M, Ung B, Kettering JD. *In vitro* bacterial penetration of coronally unsealed endodontically treated teeth. J Endod 1990;16(12):566-569. 歯冠側未封鎖の歯内治療歯の *in vitro* における細菌通過性 **本項に和訳あり**	13	8	10	8	265
引用数 3位	Wu MK, Wesselink PR. Endodontic leakage studies reconsidered. Part I. Methodology, application and relevance. Int Endod J 1993;26(1):37-43. 歯内療法における漏洩試験を再考する：1．方法、適応、および妥当性 **本項に和訳あり**	15	9	4	6	247
引用数 4位	Teixeira FB, Teixeira EC, Thompson JY, Trope M. Fracture resistance of roots endodontically treated with a new resin filling material. J Am Dent Assoc 2004;135(5):646-652. 新しいレジン系根管充填材で歯内処置された根管の破折抵抗性 **チャプター3に和訳あり**	9	14	10	9	163
引用数 5位	Shipper G, Teixeira FB, Arnold RR, Trope M. Periapical inflammation after coronal microbial inoculation of dog roots filled with gutta-percha or resilon. J Endod 2005;31(2):91-96. ガッタパーチャあるいはレジロンで根管充填したイヌ歯根における歯冠部細菌植種後の根尖性の炎症	9	5	7	6	122
引用数 6位	Meister F Jr, Lommel TJ, Gerstein H. Diagnosis and possible causes of vertical root fractures. Oral Surg Oral Med Oral Pathol 1980;49(3):243-253. 垂直性歯根破折の診断と原因 **チャプター3に和訳あり**	3	8	6	4	122

Root canal condensation

トムソン・ロイターが選んだベスト12論文

	タイトル・和訳	2011年	2012年	2013年	2014年	合計引用数
引用数 7位	Wu MK, De Gee AJ, Wesselink PR, Moorer WR. Fluid transport and bacterial penetration along root canal fillings. Int Endod J 1993；26(4)：203-208. 根管充填材に沿って生じる流体輸送と細菌通過性 **本項に和訳あり**	6	1	4	3	120
引用数 8位	Magura ME, Kafrawy AH, Brown CE Jr, Newton CW. Human saliva coronal microleakage in obturated root canals: an *in vitro* study. J Endod 1991；17(7)：324-331. 根管充填された根管におけるヒト唾液の歯冠漏洩：*in vitro* 研究 **本項に和訳あり**	6	0	4	1	120
引用数 9位	Khayat A, Lee SJ, Torabinejad M. Human saliva penetration of coronally unsealed obturated root canals. J Endod. 1993 Sep;19(9):458-61. 歯冠未封鎖根管充填歯のヒト唾液通過性	6	3	4	3	116
引用数 10位	Friedman S, Abitbol S, Lawrence HP. Treatment outcome in endodontics：the Toronto Study. Phase 1：initial treatment. J Endod 2003；29(12)：787-793. 歯内療法における治療成績：トロントスタディ．Phase 1：初期治療	7	7	4	9	90
引用数 11位	Serafino C, Gallina G, Cumbo E, Ferrari M. Surface debris of canal walls after post space preparation in endodontically treated teeth：a scanning electron microscopic study. Oral Surg Oral Med Oral Pathol Oral Radiol Endod 2004；97(3)：381-387. 根管治療歯におけるポスト形成後の根管壁表面デブリ：走査電子顕微鏡研究	9	8	11	5	76
引用数 12位	Holland R, de Souza V, Nery MJ, Otoboni Filho JA, Bernabé PF, Dezan Júnior E. Reaction of dogs' teeth to root canal filling with mineral trioxide aggregate or a glass ionomer sealer. J Endod 1999；25(11)：728-730. MTAもしくはグラスアイオノマーシーラーを用いた根管充填に対するイヌの歯の反応	5	5	3	9	76

An evaluation of microbial leakage in roots filled with a thermoplastic synthetic polymer-based root canal filling material (Resilon).

熱可塑性合成ポリマー製根管充填材（レジロン）で根管充填された歯の微小漏洩の評価

Shipper G, Ørstavik D, Teixeira FB, Trope M.

　本研究の目的は、2通りの根管充填法を用いて、ガッタパーチャと熱可塑性合成ポリマー製根管充填材（レジロン）を通過する *Streptococcus mutans* と *Enterococcus faecalis* の細菌漏洩を30日間比較することである。歯は歯冠を切除後、歯根長16mmの長さとした後、ISOサイズ40号から50号で根管形成した。計156本の歯を無作為にそれぞれ15本ずつの8グループ（グループ1～8）と3コントロールグループ（それぞれ12本ずつ）に分類した。根管は、ガッタパーチャとAH26シーラーを用いて（グループ1とグループ2）、ガッタパーチャとエピファニーシーラーを用いて（グループ3とグループ4）、それぞれ側方加圧充填法および垂直加圧充填法による根管充填を行った。レジロンとエピファニーシーラーを用いて側方加圧充填法あるいは垂直加圧充填法による根管充填を行った（グループ5とグループ6）。上部チャンバーに植菌された *Streptococcus mutans* が根管充填した根管だけを通り下部チャンバーへ到達可能な実験法の split chamber 法細菌漏洩試験が用いられた。グループ5と6と同様の充填法を行ったグループ7と8では、*E. faecalis* を漏洩試験に用いた。ポジティブコントロールは、シーラーを使用せずにレジロン（12根管）あるいはガッタパーチャ（12根管）で充填した群とし、細菌漏洩試験が行われた、一方、ネガティブコントロール（12根管）は、チャンバー間の封鎖性確認のため、ワックスで封鎖した根管とした。1例以外のすべてのポジティブコントロールが、24時間以内に細菌漏洩を生じた。一方、すべてのネガティブコントロールは漏洩を生じなかった。レジロンは最小の漏洩性を示し（グループ8：1例、グループ5～7：各2例）、根管充填法やシーラーの種類によらず試料の約80％が漏洩したガッタパーチャと比較すると有意に低かった。Kruskal-Wallis 検定を用いて、全グループ間を比較すると、統計学的有意差が認められた（$P < 0.05$）。Mann-Whitney の U 検定を用いて各グループ間を比較すると、レジロン使用群のほうがガッタパーチャ使用群より有意に封鎖性に優れていることがわかった（$P < 0.05$）。

（J Endod 2004；30（5）：342-347.）

The purpose of this study was to compare bacterial leakage using *Streptococcus mutans* and *Enterococcus faecalis* through gutta-percha and a thermoplastic synthetic polymer-based root filling (Resilon) using two filling techniques during a 30-day period. Teeth were decoronated, roots prepared to a length of 16 mm, and instrumented to ISO sizes 40 to 50. A total of 156 roots were randomly divided into 8 groups of 15 roots (groups 1-8) and 3 control groups (12 roots each). Roots were filled using lateral and vertical condensation techniques with gutta-percha and AH 26 sealer (groups 1 and 2) or with gutta-percha and Epiphany sealer (groups 3 and 4). Groups 5 and 6 were filled with Resilon and Epiphany sealer using the lateral or vertical condensation techniques. A split chamber microbial leakage model was used in which *S. mutans* placed in the upper chamber could reach the lower chamber only through the filled canal. Groups 7 and 8 were identical to groups 5 and 6 respectively; however, *E. faecalis* was used to test the leakage. Positive controls were filled with Resilon (12 roots) and gutta-percha (12 roots) without sealer and tested with bacteria, whereas negative controls (12 roots) were sealed with wax to test the seal between chambers. All but one positive control leaked within 24 h, whereas none of the negative controls leaked. Resilon showed minimal leakage (group 8 : one leakage ; groups 5-7 : each with two leakages), which was significantly less than gutta-percha, in which approximately 80% of specimens with either technique or sealer leaked. Kruskal-Wallis test showed statistical significance when all groups were compared (p<0.05). Mann-Whitney U test compared the respective groups and found Resilon groups superior to gutta-percha groups (p<0.05).

12 Root canal condensation

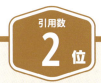

In vitro bacterial penetration of coronally unsealed endodontically treated teeth.

歯冠側未封鎖の歯内治療歯の *in vitro* における細菌通過性

Torabinejad M, Ung B, Kettering JD.

　45の根管を根管形成および根管洗浄後、側方加圧充填法を用いてガッタパーチャとシーラーで根管充填した。表皮ブドウ球菌および *Proteus vulgaris* に曝すように、歯冠部の根管充填材を配置した。これらの細菌が根管を完全に通過するのに要する日数を測定した。表皮ブドウ球菌曝露19日経過後において、試料（根管）の50％以上が完全に汚染されていた。根管充填材の歯冠部側を *Proteus vulgaris* に曝した場合でも、42日間経過すると、試料（根管）の50％以上が完全に汚染されていた。

（J Endod 1990；16（12）：566-569.）

Forty-five root canals were cleaned, shaped, and then obturated with gutta-percha and root canal sealer, using a lateral condensation technique. The coronal portions of the root filling materials were placed in contact with *Staphylococcus epidermidis* and *Proteus vulgaris*. The number of days required for these bacteria to penetrate the entire root canals was determined. Over 50% of the root canals were completely contaminated after 19-day exposure to *S. epidermidis*. Fifty percent of the root canals were also totally contaminated when the coronal surfaces of their fillings were exposed to *P. vulgaris* for 42 days.

Endodontic leakage studies reconsidered.
Part I. Methodology, application and relevance.

歯内療法における漏洩試験を再考する：
1．方法、適応、および妥当性

Wu MK, Wesselink PR.

　歯内療法学分野において、漏洩に関する研究はますます多く発表されている。Journal of Endodontics および International Endodontic Journal の1990年刊行分において、実に科学論文4.3本ごとに1本が漏洩に関する研究であった。もっとも一般的な漏洩の試験法は、根管充填材に沿って浸透した追跡子（色素や放射性同位体）の直線的距離を計測することであった。1980年から1990年までに発表された論文のうち、ガッタパーチャを用いた側方加圧充填後、色素浸透の直線的距離を測定した論文データをいくつか比べると、これらの研究に用いられた実験方法は酷似しているものの、データには大きな差異が認められた。さまざまな術式を評価したほとんどすべての漏洩研究において、側方加圧充填法が比較対象の標準コントロールとして用いられている。これらを用いた研究結果の信頼性は疑問の余地がある。そうしたことから、そのような研究の問題点が検討されている。適切な知識がほとんど得られないような実験方法で、異なる材料や術式を用いたときの封鎖性を評価し続けるよりも、漏洩試験の実験方法についてもっと研究をすべきように思える。

（Int Endod J 1993；26（1）：37-43.）

An increasing number of endodontic leakage studies have been published. In the 1990 volumes of Journal of Endodontics and International Endodontic Journal, there was one leakage study to every 4.3 scientific articles. The most popular method was linear measurement of tracer (dye or radioisotope) penetration along a root filling. Comparing some data on linear measurement of dye penetration following the cold lateral condensation of gutta-percha that were published between 1980 and 1990, a high level of variation has been found, although the experimental methods used in these studies were quite similar. In almost all studies evaluating various techniques, the cold lateral condensation technique has been used as a standard control for comparison. The reliability of these results is questionable. The problems with such studies are discussed. It seems that more research should be done on leakage study methodology, instead of continuing to evaluate the sealing ability of different materials and techniques by methods that may give little relevant information.

Fluid transport and bacterial penetration along root canal fillings.

根管充填材に沿って生じる流体輸送と細菌通過性

Wu MK, De Gee AJ, Wesselink PR, Moorer WR.

　根管充填した根管の歯冠側から根尖までの水の対流搬送は、120 kPa（1.2気圧）のヘッドスペース圧を用いて実験的歯根片の根尖につないだガラス毛細管内の気泡の移動から測定した。根管充填した根管内に生じた死腔を通過した水の移動は、前述の方法で再現性ある測定が可能であるとわかった。60歯のヒト上顎犬歯歯根を、側方加圧充填法でガッタパーチャとシーラーを用いて根管充填した。このうち30歯に、まず、歯根の歯冠側のレゼルボア（病原巣）において増殖させた小運動性細菌の緑膿菌を暴露した。50日後、2つの試料で根尖側レゼルボアへの細菌通過を認めた。そして、すべての根管は、水の対流搬送の定量評価に供された。評価結果は、以下の"細菌漏洩性がない"（39根管）、"わずかな細菌漏洩"（14根管）、および"著しい細菌漏洩"（7根管）という3つの明確なカテゴリーに分類された。根尖側レゼルボアへの細菌通過が認められた2つの試料は、1つは"わずかな細菌漏洩"、そして、もう1つは"著しい細菌漏洩"のカテゴリーに分類された。既往の細菌通過試験では、実験後の計測におけるこれら歯根の液体流動パターンに統計学的な影響を認めなかった。これらの所見は、根管充填された根管における流体移動においては、その根管のほとんどで細菌通過を認めないことを示している。

（Int Endod J 1993；26（4）：203-208.）

Convective transport of water from the coronal to the apical end of obturated root canals was determined by the movement of an air bubble in a capillary glass tube connected to the apex of the experimental root section using a headspace pressure of 120 kPa (1.2 atm). Water transport through existing voids in the obturated canals could be measured reproducibly in this way. The root canals of 60 human maxillary canines were filled with gutta-percha and sealer by the cold lateral condensation technique. Thirty of these were first exposed to a small motile bacterium, *Pseudomonas aeruginosa*, growing in a reservoir at the coronal end of each root. After 50 days, two specimens allowed penetration of bacteria to a reservoir at the apical end. All the roots were then assessed quantitatively for convective transport of water. The results were divided into three defined categories: 39 obturated canals were in the "bacteria tight" category, 14 canals in the "slight leakage" and 7 canals in the "gross leakage" category. The two specimens that showed bacterial penetration fell into the slight and gross leakage categories. The previous test for bacterial passage did not statistically influence the fluid transport pattern of these roots which was measured subsequently. These findings indicate that fluids transport through obturated root canals, most of which do not allow the passage of bacteria.

引用数
8位

Human saliva coronal microleakage in obturated root canals：an *in vitro* study.

根管充填された根管におけるヒト唾液の歯冠漏洩：*in vitro* 研究

Magura ME，Kafrawy AH，Brown CE Jr，Newton CW.

本研究は、組織学的検索と色素浸透の２つの手法を用いて、根管充填された根管の唾液浸透を時間的に評価することである。総計160本のヒト上顎前歯が60号のＨファイルで根管形成された。それらの歯のうち10歯は根管充填を行わず、そして150歯はガッタパーチャとRothのシーラーによる側方加圧充填法を用いた根管充填が行われた。50歯は、厚さ約３mmとなるように仮封材を充填した。すべての歯はヒト全唾液50mL中に浸漬し、湿度100%、温度37℃で保存した。唾液は毎日交換した。２日、７日、14日、28日、90日ごとに、32歯を唾液から取りだした。これらのうち２歯は根管充填をしない歯とし、根尖部1/3を培養することにより細菌漏洩を検索した。未仮封の10歯は、唾液浸透範囲を明らかにするために、ペリカンインクに２日間浸漬した。これらの歯は、脱灰後、色素浸透範囲を直接測定できるように透明標本にした。残り20歯（仮封歯10歯と未仮封歯10歯）から、厚さ７μmの脱灰連続切片を作成した。切片はヘマトキシリン・エオジン染色とグラム染色（Brown-Hopps 染色）を行った。組織切片において評価された唾液浸透は、色素分析で可視化された唾液浸透より有意に小さかった。３か月後の唾液浸透は、３か月以前の４つの観察期間と比べて有意に大きかった。この唾液浸透量は臨床的意義を有すると考えられた。今回の結果は、少なくとも３か月間口腔内に曝露されると根管充填された根管でも再治療すべきであることを強く示唆している。

（J Endod 1991；17（７）：324-331.）

This study assessed salivary penetration through obturated root canals as related to time by using two methods of analysis-histological examination and dye penetrations. A total of 160 human maxillary anterior teeth were instrumented to size 60 Hedstrom file. Ten of the teeth were not obturated; 150 teeth were obturated by lateral condensation of gutta-percha and Roth's root canal sealer. Fifty of these teeth received intermediate restorative material temporaries to a thickness of approximately 3mm. All teeth were immersed in 50 ml of whole human saliva and kept at 37 degrees C and 100% humidity. The saliva was changed daily. At 2, 7, 14, 28, and 90 days, 32 teeth were removed from the saliva. Of these, two were unobturated and were examined for bacterial penetration by culturing of the apical one-third. Ten teeth without temporaries were immersed in Pelikan ink for 2 days to demonstrate the extent of salivary penetration. These teeth were decalcified and cleared to allow direct measurement of dye penetration. Decalcified serial 7-microns-thick sections were prepared from the remaining 20 teeth, 10 with and 10 without intermediate restorative material temporaries. The sections were stained with hematoxylin and eosin stain and Brown and Hopps stain. Saliva penetration assessed in histological sections was significantly less than was visualized with dye analysis. Salivary penetration at 3 months was significantly greater than at the four earlier study periods. This amount of salivary penetration was considered to be clinically significant. The results strongly suggest retreatment of obturated root canals that have been exposed to the oral cavity for at least 3 months.

エンドのための重要20キーワード

13 *Microleakage*

微小漏洩

根管充填による十分な根管封鎖性が得られず、根尖歯周組織へ細菌や細菌関連物質などの微小漏洩が生じてしまうと、予後不良となることがある。そのため、緊密でよりよい封鎖性の根管充填を達成することを目的として多数の研究が行われている。また、歯内治療時の仮封材、外科的歯内療法での逆根管充填材、そして穿孔部の封鎖材においても、同様に歯内療法の予後を左右することから、種々の報告が行われている。

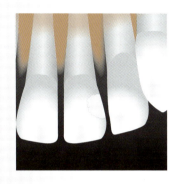

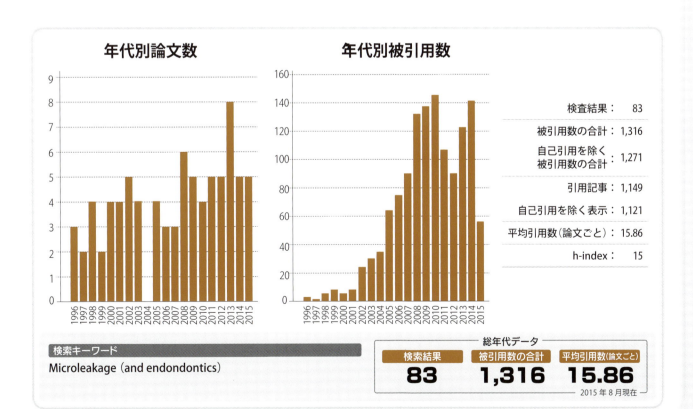

検索キーワード: Microleakage (and endondontics)

検査結果: 83
被引用数の合計: 1,316
自己引用を除く被引用数の合計: 1,271
引用記事: 1,149
自己引用を除く表示: 1,121
平均引用数(論文ごと): 15.86
h-index: 15

総年代データ
検索結果: 83
被引用数の合計: 1,316
平均引用数(論文ごと): 15.86
2015年8月現在

トムソン・ロイターが選んだベスト12論文

	タイトル・和訳	2011年	2012年	2013年	2014年	合計引用数
引用数 1位	Torabinejad M, Chivian N. Clinical applications of mineral trioxide aggregate. J Endod 1999；25（3）：197-205. **Mineral trioxide aggregate の臨床応用** チャプター16に和訳あり	36	31	31	42	406
引用数 2位	Torabinejad M, Handysides R, Khademi AA, Bakland LK. Clinical implications of the smear layer in endodontics：a review. Oral Surg Oral Med Oral Pathol Oral Radiol Endod 2002；94（6）：658-666. **歯内療法におけるスメアー層の臨床的意味：総説論文** チャプター9に和訳あり	15	8	12	17	160
引用数 3位	Roberts HW, Toth JM, Berzins DW, Charlton DG. Mineral trioxide aggregate material use in endodontic treatment：a review of the literature. Dent Mater 2008；24（2）：149-164. **歯内療法における mineral trioxide aggregate 材料の使用：文献展望**	20	13	21	21	127
引用数 4位	Ricucci D, Bergenholtz G. Bacterial status in root-filled teeth exposed to the oral environment by loss of restoration and fracture or caries — a histobacteriological study of treated cases. Int Endod J 2003；36(11)：787-802. **修復物の喪失および破折、あるいはう蝕により口腔内環境に暴露された根管充填歯の細菌状態―治療症例の組織細菌学的研究** 本項に和訳あり	7	4	13	5	65
引用数 5位	Bobotis HG, Anderson RW, Pashley DH, Pantera EA Jr. A microleakage study of temporary restorative materials used in endodontics. J Endod 1989；15(12)：569-572. **歯内療法に用いられる仮封材の微小漏洩研究** 本項に和訳あり	0	1	2	0	40
引用数 6位	Pommel L, Camps J. Effects of pressure and measurement time on the fluid filtration method in endodontics. J Endod 2001；27（4）：256-258. **歯内療法における流体移動法に対する圧力および測定時間の影響**	1	2	4	0	34

13 Microleakage

トムソン・ロイターが選んだベスト**12**論文

	タイトル・和訳	2011年	2012年	2013年	2014年	合計引用数
引用数 **7**位	Martell B, Chandler NP. Electrical and dye leakage comparison of three root-end restorative materials. Quintessence Int 2002；33（1）：30-34. 3種の逆根管充填材の電気的漏洩試験および色素漏洩試験による比較 **本項に和訳あり**	0	3	1	0	34
引用数 **8**位	De Bruyne MA, De Bruyne RJ, Rosiers L, De Moor RJ. Longitudinal study on microleakage of three root-end filling materials by the fluid transport method and by capillary flow porometry. Int Endod J 2005；38（2）：129-136. 流体移動法およびキャピラリーフローポロメトリー法による3種の逆根管充填材の微小漏洩に対する長期的研究 **本項に和訳あり**	3	0	2	1	34
引用数 **9**位	Gomes BP, Sato E, Ferraz CC, Teixeira FB, Zaia AA, Souza-Filho FJ. Evaluation of time required for recontamination of coronally sealed canals medicated with calcium hydroxide and chlorhexidine. Int Endod J 2003；36（9）：604-609. 水酸化カルシウムとクロルヘキシジンを貼薬し、歯冠側を仮封した根管が再感染するまでに要する時間の評価	0	2	4	3	29
引用数 **10**位	Niemiec BA. Fundamentals of endodontics. Vet Clin North Am Small Anim Pract 2005；35（4）：837-868. 歯内療法の基本	4	2	3	2	21
引用数 **11**位	Naoum HJ, Chandler NP. Temporization for endodontics. Int Endod J 2002；35(12)：964-978. 歯内療法における仮封	0	2	2	2	21
引用数 **12**位	Jacquot BM, Panighi MM, Steinmetz P, G'sell C. Evaluation of temporary restorations' microleakage by means of electrochemical impedance measurements. J Endod 1996；22(11)：586-589. 電気的インピーダンス測定による仮封材の微小漏洩の評価	2	2	0	1	17

Bacterial status in root-filled teeth exposed to the oral environment by loss of restoration and fracture or caries — a histobacteriological study of treated cases.

修復物の喪失および破折、あるいはう蝕により口腔内環境に暴露された根管充填歯の細菌状態―治療症例の組織細菌学的研究

Ricucci D, Bergenholtz G.

目的：根管充填材が長期間う蝕や口腔内環境に暴露された歯の組織学的ならびに細菌学的所見について説明すること。

方法：本研究の検索対象歯として、少なくとも3か月以上適切な修復処置が施されず、さらに3年以上の予後観察をした根管充填歯のみを選択した。そのうちの何本かは、数年間、修復処置をされていなかった。32歯の39根管を組織学的に検索した。

結果：検索歯の大部分は、エックス線評価において、明白な根尖病変を認めなかった。溶骨性病変は5根管に観察された。改良型Brown/Bren染色を用いて染色した歯根長軸方向の組織切片では、根管口や根管口部の象牙細管内には多量の染色液陽性の細菌が観察されたが、2歯を除くすべての試料において根中央部および根尖側では細菌が観察されなかった。39根管中7根管において細菌侵入があったことを示唆する所見である根尖部軟組織および根尖分枝内の明瞭な炎症性細胞浸潤が認められた。この7根管以外の全試料において、炎症性細胞浸潤は認められないか、散在している程度で、これらの散在性の細胞浸潤は、溢出したシーラー材料に関連したものであった。

結論：質の高い根管形成と根管充填が施された根管は、う蝕、あるいは修復物の喪失や破折により長期間口腔内環境に暴露されたとしても、細菌通過性に対して抵抗性を有する。

(Int Endod J 2003；36(11)：787-802.)

AIM: To describe histological and microbiological findings in teeth where root fillings had been exposed to caries and the oral environment for a prolonged period.
METHODOLOGY: For inclusion in the study, only teeth with a follow-up period of 3 years or more and those that had been without proper restoration for at least a period of 3 months were considered. Some root fillings had been without restoration for several years. In all, 39 roots representing 32 teeth were examined by histology.
RESULTS: The majority of the specimens were without a discernible periapical bone lesion as assessed by radiography. Osteolytic lesions were seen with five roots. Longitudinal tissue sections stained with a modified Brown/Brenn staining technique revealed presence of stainable bacteria in abundance at the canal entrance and in dentinal tubules but were absent mid-root and apically in all but two specimens. Soft tissue attached to the root tip and in apical ramifications displayed distinct inflammatory cell infiltrates, suggesting microbial exposure in 7 of the 39 roots examined. In all other specimens, inflammatory cell infiltrates were either nonexistent or sparse and then associated with extruded sealer material.
CONCLUSIONS: Well-prepared and filled root canals resist bacterial penetration even upon frank and long-standing oral exposure by caries, fracture or loss of restoration.

Microleakage

A microleakage study of temporary restorative materials used in endodontics.

歯内療法に用いられる仮封材の微小漏洩研究

Bobotis HG, Anderson RW, Pashley DH, Pantera EA Jr.

　本研究の目的は、新規に導入した流体濾過法を用いて、一般の歯内療法に用いられる種々の仮封材の封鎖性を定量評価することである。その評価材料としてCavit、Cavit-G、TERM、グラスアイオノマーセメント、リン酸亜鉛セメント、ポリカルボキシレートセメント、およびIRMを用いた。ヒト切歯、犬歯、および小臼歯の抜去歯を検索対象とし、そしてそれらに対して髄腔開拡を行う前に漏洩試験を行うことで各検索歯に対する同一対照（コントロール）とした。髄腔開拡後、綿球を髄腔内に置き、仮封材の厚みを4mmとした。仮封後、ただちに検索歯はリンガー液に浸漬され、37℃の恒温で放置された。漏洩は、さまざまに時間間隔を設定して測定した。観察期間8週間を通して、Cavit、Cavit-G、TERM、グラスアイオノマーセメントはこの漏洩試験に耐えうる封鎖材と考えられたが、一方、リン酸亜鉛セメントによる仮封では10歯のうち4歯に漏洩が観察された。IRMとポリカルボン酸セメントは、漏洩試験した材料のなかでもっとも封鎖性に対する効果の乏しい材料であった。

(J Endod 1989; 15(12): 569-572.)

The purpose of this study was to quantitatively evaluate the sealing properties of various temporary restorative materials used in standard endodontic access preparations by using a newly introduced fluid filtration method. The materials tested were Cavit, Cavit-G, TERM, glass ionomer cement, zinc phosphate cement, polycarboxylate cement, and IRM. Extracted human incisor, canine, and premolar teeth were used, and each tooth served as its own control by testing for microleakage prior to access preparation. Following access preparation, cotton pellets were placed in the pulp chamber so that the space remaining for the restoration was 4 mm. Immediately after placement of the restoration, the teeth were immersed in Ringer's solution and incubated at 37 degrees C. Microleakage was measured after various time intervals. The results indicated that Cavit, Cavit-G, TERM, and glass ionomer cement provided leakproof seals during the 8-wk testing period, while leakage was observed in 4 of the 10 teeth restored with zinc phosphate cement. IRM and polycarboxylate cement were the least effective of the materials tested for preventing microleakage.

Electrical and dye leakage comparison of three root-end restorative materials.

3種の逆根管充填材の電気的漏洩試験および色素漏洩試験による比較

Martell B, Chandler NP.

目的：本研究の目的は、電気的漏洩試験法と色素浸透漏洩試験法により、近年使用されている3種類の逆根管充填材の評価をすることである。

方法と材料：33本のヒト犬歯は根管形成後、ガッタパーチャとシーラーを用いて根管充填された。電極として根管にステンレススチール製の棒を挿入し、そして歯の表面にワニス（varnish）を塗布した。それぞれの歯の根尖から3mmで根尖部を切除した後、超音波を用いて3mmの深さで逆根管窩洞形成を行った。MTA、Super EBA、IRM を用い、それぞれ10歯に逆根管充填した。そしてワニス塗布のみの3歯をコントロールとした。血液中に24時間置いた後、試料は1％塩化カリウム電解液中に置かれた。そして観察期間を70日間として漏洩を電気的に測定した。その後、歯をメチレンブルー染色液中に72時間浸漬し、長軸方向に薄切した後、6名の試験者による色素漏洩の評価を行った。

結果：両試験法において、MTA 充填は IRM や Super EBA 充填に比較して有意に低い漏洩性を示した。電気的漏洩試験において、Super EBA 充填は IRM 充填に比べて有意に低い漏洩性を示したが、色素浸透試験においては両者に有意差は認められなかった。MTA で封鎖した歯は、ワニスを塗布したネガティブコントロール歯と同様の封鎖性を示した。

結論：本研究結果は、MTA が逆根管充填材として優れた封鎖性を有することを示唆した。

（Quintessence Int 2002；33（1）：30-34.）

OBJECTIVE: The purpose of this study was to assess three modern root-end restorative materials with electrical and dye leakage tests.
METHOD AND MATERIALS: Thirty-three human canine teeth were prepared and filled with gutta-percha and sealer. Stainless steel rods were inserted into the root canals as anodes, and the teeth were varnished. The apical 3 mm of each tooth was resected, and 3-mm root-end preparations were made ultrasonically. Mineral trioxide aggregate, Super EBA, and IRM were used to restore 10 teeth each, and three teeth were varnished as controls. Following 24 hours' setting in blood, the specimens were placed in 1% potassium chloride electrolyte, and leakage was recorded electrically for 70 days. The teeth were then submerged in methylene blue dye for 72 hours, sectioned longitudinally, and scored for leakage by six examiners.
RESULTS: In both tests, the mineral trioxide aggregate restorations leaked significantly less than the IRM and Super EBA restorations. Super EBA showed significantly less leakage than did IRM restorations in the electrochemical test but not in the dye leakage experiment. The teeth sealed with mineral trioxide aggregate performed similarly to the varnished negative control teeth.
CONCLUSION: The results of this study indicated that mineral trioxide aggregate provides a superior seal in root-end-restorations.

Longitudinal study on microleakage of three root-end filling materials by the fluid transport method and by capillary flow porometry.

流体移動法およびキャピラリーフローポロメトリー法による
3種の逆根管充填材の微小漏洩に対する長期的研究

De Bruyne MA, De Bruyne RJ, Rosiers L, De Moor RJ.

目的：(1)逆根管充填材である IRM Caps(IRM)、Fuji IX Capsules(Fuji IX)、Pro Root MTA Tooth-Coloured Formula(MTA)の根端部根管封鎖性を、屍体から得られた歯を用いて比較すること。(2)流体移動法とキャピラリーフローポロメトリー法(CFP)を比較することにより、漏洩試験の方法に対するさらなる検索を行うこと。　方法：歯根端切除と超音波チップ(Suni-Max製 S12/90°D-tip)によって逆根管形成した歯を採取するための前処置として、その2週間前に、屍体33体の生体位において歯内療法が行われた。2歯は陽性対照および陰性対照とした。それ以外の歯は、無作為に3群に分類された後、3種の逆根管充填材のいずれかをそれぞれ充填した。逆根管充填材は、充填後5分間水に曝された。根管充填材を根管内から除去した後、それぞれの歯は37℃で12時間保管された。それらの漏洩量L(μL/日)は、流体移動法を用いて1.2気圧下にて24時間計測し、そしてL＝0、0＜L≦10、L＞10のいずれかとして記録した。この測定は逆根管充填から1か月後と6か月後も繰り返し行われた。6か月後においては、逆根管充填材を貫いて根尖へ開口している細孔数とその細孔の半径を計測するため、キャピラリーフローポロメトリー法を用いての漏洩の評価も行われた。実験結果はノンパラメトリック法である Kruskal-Wallis 検定および Mann–Whitney U 検定を用いて、両検定法の結果の相関は、スピアマンの順位相関係数を用いて算出した。有意水準は0.05とした。　結果：(1)流体移動法を用いた1か月における評価では、FujiIX と IRM の間に統計学的有意差が認められた。6か月において、流体移動法による評価では、FujiIX とそれ以外の材料との間には統計学的有意差が認められたが、キャピラリーフローポロメトリー法による評価では有意差は認められなかった。しかしながら、どちらの試験法を用いても、FujiIX がもっとも良好な封鎖性を示していた。(2) 2つの漏洩試験法を比較すると、キャピラリーフローポロメトリー法では逆根管充填材を貫いて根尖に開口している細孔をすべての歯において確認できたが、一方、流体移動法では31歯中14歯だけしか、根尖まで開口している細孔を確認できなかった。両者の漏洩試験法には正の相関関係が認められた。　結論：本研究の実験条件下においては、(1)グラスアイオノマーセメント FujiIX は逆根管充填材として使用したときにもっとも良好な結果を示した。(2)キャピラリーフローポロメトリー法は、歯内療法における材料を貫いて開口しているような細孔に対する漏洩評価に有効な試験法であると考えられた。

(Int Endod J 2005；38(2)：129-136.)

AIM: (i) To compare the root-end sealing ability of IRM Caps (IRM). Fuji IX Capsules (Fuji IX) and Pro Root MTA Tooth-Coloured Formula (MTA) in teeth obtained from cadavers. (ii) Further research on leakage study methodology by means of comparison of the fluid transport method (FTM) and capillary flow porometry (CFP).
METHODOLOGY: Root canal treatment was performed on 33 cadaver teeth in situ 2 weeks prior to root resection and ultrasonic retropreparation (S12/90 degrees D-tip on Suni-Max), after which the teeth were retrieved from the cadavers. Two teeth were kept as positive and negative controls. The other teeth were divided in three different groups at random, with each group receiving one of the retrofill materials. Retrofills were exposed to water 5 min after placement. The teeth were stored at 37 degrees C for 12 h after which the root filling was removed. Microleakage (L in microL day (-1)) was measured for 24 h under a pressure of 1.2 atm using FTM and recorded as L=0, 0<L<or=10, L>10. The measurements were repeated after 1 and 6 months. After 6 months, leakage was also assessed by CFP in order to measure through pores and their diameters. Results were analysed statistically using nonparametric Kruskal-Wallis and Mann-Whitney U-tests, and Spearman correlation coefficients between the results of both methods were calculated. The level of significance was set at 0.05.
RESULTS: (i) A statistically significant difference could be demonstrated between Fuji IX and IRM at 1 month with FTM. FTM revealed a significant difference between Fuji IX and the other materials at 6 months, whereas CFP did not. However, using both methods, Fuji IX showed the best result. (ii) When comparing both techniques, CFP demonstrated through pores in all teeth, whereas with FTM in only 14 of the 31 teeth could through pores be demonstrated. A positive correlation between both methods was demonstrated.
CONCLUSIONS; Under the conditions of this study (i) the conventionally setting glass-ionomer cement Fuji IX showed the best results when used as a root-end material and (ii) CFP appeared to be a useful method for leakage evaluation of through pores in endodontics.

エンドのための重要20キーワード

14 Endodontic microsurgery
マイクロサージェリー

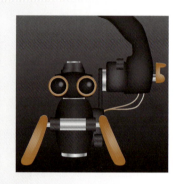

医療器具としての実体顕微鏡の歴史は、1922年にストックホルム大学のCral Nylenが耳の外科処置に単眼の顕微鏡を用いたことに始まった。そのおよそ30年後の1953年に、Carl Zeiss社が双眼の医科用実体顕微鏡を商品化した。それ以降、実体顕微鏡はさまざまな医療分野に導入されていく。歯科における実体顕微鏡(Dental operating microscope)の導入は、ハーバード大学歯学部のApothekerらにより、1978年に初めて行われた。その後、1993年に、歯科用実体顕微鏡による外科的歯内療法の最初のシンポジウムがペンシルバニア大学において開催され、その重要性が再認識され始めて以降、欧米を中心に広まっていくことになる。

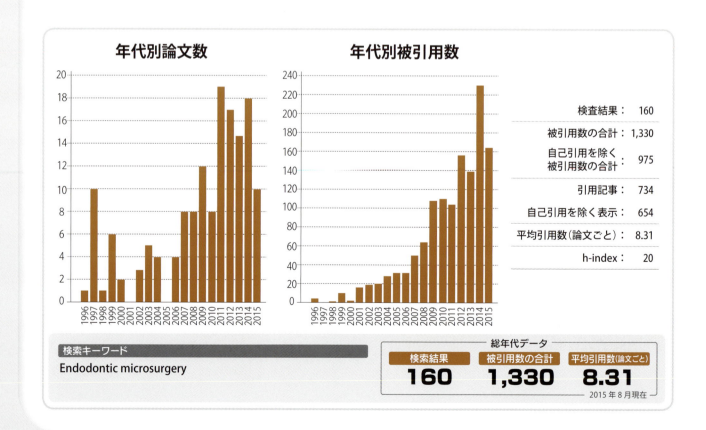

検索キーワード: Endodontic microsurgery

検査結果	160
被引用数の合計	1,330
自己引用を除く被引用数の合計	975
引用記事	734
自己引用を除く表示	654
平均引用数(論文ごと)	8.31
h-index	20

総年代データ
- 検索結果: 160
- 被引用数の合計: 1,330
- 平均引用数(論文ごと): 8.31

2015年8月現在

⑭ Endodontic microsurgery

トムソン・ロイターが選んだベスト12論文

	タイトル・和訳	2011年	2012年	2013年	2014年	合計引用数
引用数 1位	Kim S, Kratchman S. Modern endodontic surgery concepts and practice：a review. J Endod 2006；32(7)：601-623. 近代的外科的歯内療法の概念と診療：総説論文 **本項に和訳あり**	20	20	10	21	136
引用数 2位	Kim E, Song JS, Jung IY, Lee SJ, Kim S. Prospective clinical study evaluating endodontic microsurgery outcomes for cases with lesions of endodontic origin compared with cases with lesions of combined periodontal-endodontic origin. J Endod 2008；34(5)：546-551. 外科的歯内療法後の予後評価においてエンド・ペリオ病変を併発した症例と歯内病変を有する症例とを比較した前向き臨床研究 **本項に和訳あり**	4	6	7	9	40
引用数 3位	Setzer FC, Shah SB, Kohli MR, Karabucak B, Kim S. Outcome of endodontic surgery：a meta-analysis of the literature — part 1：Comparison of traditional root-end surgery and endodontic microsurgery. J Endod 2010；36(11)：1757-1765. 外科的歯内療法の治療成果：文献のメタ解析—Part 1：従来法による歯根端切除術とエンドドンティック・マイクロサージェリーとの比較 **本項に和訳あり**	5	6	7	11	36
引用数 4位	Gu L, Wei X, Ling J, Huang X. A microcomputed tomographic study of canal isthmuses in the mesial root of mandibular first molars in a Chinese population. J Endod 2009；35(3)：353-356. 中国人の下顎第一大臼歯近心根における根管イスムスのマイクロトモグラフィによる研究 **本項に和訳あり**	4	4	3	3	27
引用数 5位	von Arx T, Jensen SS, Hänni S, Friedman S. Five-year longitudinal assessment of the prognosis of apical microsurgery. J Endod 2012；38(5)：570-579. 根尖部マイクロサージェリーの予後に関する5年の長期評価 **本項に和訳あり**	0	1	7	9	26
引用数 6位	Setzer FC, Kohli MR, Shah SB, Karabucak B, Kim S. Outcome of endodontic surgery：a meta-analysis of the literature — Part 2：Comparison of endodontic microsurgical techniques with and without the use of higher magnification. J Endod 2012；38(1)：1-10. 外科的歯内療法の予後：文献のメタ解析—Part 2：顕微鏡の技術を用いた手術と顕微鏡を用いない手術の比較	0	2	4	11	23

トムソン・ロイターが選んだベスト**12**論文

	タイトル・和訳	2011年	2012年	2013年	2014年	合計引用数
引用数 7位	Metska ME, Aartman IH, Wesselink PR, Özok AR. Detection of vertical root fractures *in vivo* in endodontically treated teeth by cone-beam computed tomography scans. J Endod 2012；38(10)：1344-1347. コーンビームCTによる根管治療歯の垂直性歯根破折の *in vivo* における検出率	0	0	4	11	21
引用数 8位	Song M, Jung IY, Lee SJ, Lee CY, Kim E. Prognostic factors for clinical outcomes in endodontic microsurgery：a retrospective study. J Endod 2011；37(7)：927-933. 外科的歯内療法の臨床成績の予後因子：後向き研究	1	5	5	4	18
引用数 9位	Samara A, Sarri Y, Stravopodis D, Tzanetakis GN, Kontakiotis EG, Anastasiadou E. A comparative study of the effects of three root-end filling materials on proliferation and adherence of human periodontal ligament fibroblasts. J Endod 2011；37(6)：865-870. 3種の逆根管充填材がヒト歯根膜線維芽細胞の増殖と付着に及ぼす影響の比較試験	0	4	1	9	17
引用数 10位	Bird DC, Komabayashi T, Guo L, Opperman LA, Spears R. *In vitro* evaluation of dentinal tubule penetration and biomineralization ability of a new root-end filling material. J Endod 2012；38(8)：1093-1096. 新しい逆根管充填材の象牙細管浸透能と生物による硬組織形成(biomineralization)能の *in vitro* における評価	0	0	4	5	13
引用数 11位	Song M, Shin SJ, Kim E. Outcomes of endodontic micro-resurgery：a prospective clinical study. J Endod 2011；37(3)：316-320. エンドドンティック・マイクロサージェリーの治療成果：前向き臨床研究	2	4	1	1	12
引用数 12位	Creasy JE, Mines P, Sweet M. Surgical trends among endodontists：the results of a web-based survey. J Endod 2009；35(1)：30-34. 歯内療法における外科的動向：ウェブ調査の結果	2	1	0	2	11

Modern endodontic surgery concepts and practice : a review.

近代的外科的歯内療法の概念と診療：総説論文

Kim S, Kratchman S.

　外科的歯内療法は、今やエンドドンティック・マイクロサージェリーへと進化した。生物学的概念と臨床とが対応した最先端の設備、器具および材料を用いた顕微鏡手術の導入は歯内由来病変治癒における確実な治療効果を生むと考えられる。この総説において、マイクロサージェリーがどこまで到達しているかを説明するために、最新の概念、技法、器具および材料について示したい。われわれの最終目的は次世代の大学院生に自信をもって指導すること、歯内専門医にマイクロサージェリーの技術と概念を日常の臨床に活用できるように養成することである。

（J Endod 2006；32（7）：601-623.）

Endodontic surgery has now evolved into endodontic microsurgery. By using state-of-the-art equipment, instruments and materials that match biological concepts with clinical practicem, we believe that microsurgical approaches produce predictable outcomes in the healing of lesions of endodontic origin. In this review we attempted to provide the most current conceptsm, techniques, instruments and materials with the aim of demonstrating how far we have come. Our ultimate goal is to assertively teach the future generation of graduate students and also train our colleagues to incorporate these techniques and concepts into everyday practice.

Prospective clinical study evaluating endodontic microsurgery outcomes for cases with lesions of endodontic origin compared with cases with lesions of combined periodontal-endodontic origin.

外科的歯内療法後の予後評価においてエンド・ペリオ病変を併発した症例と歯内病変を有する症例とを比較した前向き臨床研究

Kim E, Song JS, Jung IY, Lee SJ, Kim S.

　本研究の目的は、エンド・ペリオ病変の症例と歯内病変の症例を比較することで、エンドドンティック・マイクロサージェリーの治療成績を評価することである。2001年3月〜2005年6月の間に韓国・ソウル市の延世大学歯科部保存学講座に来院した患者から試料は収集された。外科的歯内療法を必要とする227名の患者の263本の歯を本研究の検索対象とした。臨床所見とエックス線写真所見による治癒評価をするため、最初の2年は6か月ごとに、それ以降は1年ごとに、患者のリコールを行った。リコール率は73％（263名中192名）であった。歯内単独病変における成功率は95.2％であった。一方、エンド・ペリオ合併病変における成功率は77.5％であった。このことは、病変のタイプ（ABC対DEF）が、組織および骨治癒に強い影響を及ぼしていることを示唆している。

（J Endod 2008；34（5）：546-551.）

The aim of this study was to evaluate the outcomes of endodontic microsurgery by comparing the healing success of cases having a lesion of endodontic origin compared with cases having a lesion of combined endodontic-periodontal origin. Data were collected from patients in the Department of Conservative Dentistry, Dental College, Yonsei University, Seoul, Korea between March 2001 and June 2005. A total number of 263 teeth from 227 patients requiring periradicular surgery were included in this study. Patients were recalled every 6 months for 2 years and every year thereafter to assess clinical and radiographic signs of healing. A recall rate of 73% (192 of 263 patients) was obtained. The successful outcome for isolated endodontic lesions was 95.2%. In endodontic-periodontal combined lesions, successful outcome was 77.5%, suggesting that lesion type (ABC vs DEF) had a strong effect on tissue and bone healing.

Endodontic microsurgery

Outcome of endodontic surgery : a meta-analysis of the literature — Part 1 : Comparison of traditional root-end surgery and endodontic microsurgery.

外科的歯内療法の治療成果：文献のメタ解析— Part 1：従来法による歯根端切除術とエンドドンティック・マイクロサージェリーとの比較

Setzer FC, Shah SB, Kohli MR, Karabucak B, Kim S.

緒言：本研究の目的は歯根端切除術の治療成績を検索することである。従来法を用いた歯根端切除術とエンドドンティック・マイクロサージェリーの特徴的な治療結果、および比較対象であるこの2つの手技の成功率を、文献のメタ解析と系統的レビューという手法を用いることにより、明確にすることである。

方法：歯根端切除術の治療成績を評価した縦断的研究を特定するため、集約的な文献検索が行われた。3つの電子データベース(Medline、Embase、およびPubMed)において、1966年から2009年10月までの間に発表されたヒトを検索対象とした研究のうち5言語(英語、フランス語、ドイツ語、イタリア語、スペイン語)で書かれた研究を検索した。関連論文や総説論文は相互参照して検索した。5つの外科的歯内療法に関連する雑誌(Journal of Endodontics、International Endodontic Journal、Oral Surgery Oral Medicine Oral Pathology Oral Radiology and Endodontics、Journal of Oral and Maxillofacial Surgery、International Journal of Oral and Maxillofacial Surgery)は、個別に1975年まで遡って検索した。3名の査読者は別個に所定の適格基準と除外基準に従って検索されたすべての論文要旨を審査した。関連論文は全文形式で取り込まれた後、生データが各査読者によって別個に抽出された。適格基準を満たしている論文はTRSもしくはEMSのどちらかのグループに振り分けられた。TRSとEMS間のウエイトづき成功率と相対危険度評価が算出された。両グループ間の比較はランダム効果モデルによって行われた。

結果：98本の論文が特定され、そして最終解析が行われた。適格基準と除外基準により、合計で21論文(そのうち12論文がTRSグループ(n＝925)、そして9論文のEMSグループ(n＝699))が選択された。抽出した生データから算出したウエイトづき成功率はTRSに対する前向きな結果(positive outocome)は59％(95％信頼区間、0.55-0.6308)、EMSで94％(95％信頼区間、0.8889-0.9816)であった。両者間には、統計学的有意差な有意差($P < .0005$)が認められた。EMSの成功確率はTRSの1.58倍ということを相対危険度は示していた。

結論：歯根端切除術において、マイクロサージェリーのテクニックを用いることは、従来のテクニックを用いることに比べて、予見される成功率はさらに優位なものとなる。

(J Endod 2010；36(11)：1757-1765.)

INTRODUCTION: The aim of this study was to investigate the outcome of root-end surgery. The specific outcome of traditional root-end surgery (TRS) versus endodontic microsurgery (EMS) and the probability of success for comparison of the 2 techniques were determined by means of meta-analysis and systematic review of the literature.
METHODS: An intensive search of the literature was conducted to identify longitudinal studies evaluating the outcome of root-end surgery. Three electronic databases (Medline, Embase, and PubMed) were searched to identify human studies from 1966 to October 2009 in 5 different languages (English, French, German, Italian, and Spanish). Relevant articles and review papers were searched for cross-references. Five pertinent journals (Journal of Endodontics, International Endodontic Journal, Oral Surgery Oral Medicine Oral Pathology Oral Radiology and Endodontics, Journal of Oral and Maxillofacial Surgery, International Journal of Oral and Maxillofacial Surgery) were individually searched back to 1975. Three independent reviewers (S.S., M.K., and F.S.) assessed the abstracts of all articles that were found according to predefined inclusion and exclusion criteria. Relevant articles were acquired in full-text form, and raw data were extracted independently by each reviewer. Qualifying papers were assigned to group TRS or group EMS. Weighted pooled success rates and relative risk assessment between TRS and EMS were calculated. A comparison between the groups was made by using a random effects model.
RESULTS: Ninety-eight articles were identified and obtained for final analysis. In total, 21 studies qualified (12 for TRS [n=925] and 9 for EMS [n=699] according to the inclusion and exclusion criteria. Weighted pooled success rates calculated from extracted raw data showed 59% positive outcome for TRS (95% confidence interval, 0.55-0.6308)and 94% for EMS (95% confidence interval, 0.8889-0.9816). This difference was statistically significant (P<.0005). The relative risk ratio showed that the probability of success for EMS was 1.58 times the probability of success for TRS.
CONCLUSIONS: The use of microsurgical techniques is superior in achieving predictably high success rates for root-end surgery when compared with traditional techniques.

A microcomputed tomographic study of canal isthmuses in the mesial root of mandibular first molars in a Chinese population.

中国人の下顎第一大臼歯近心根における根管イスムスのマイクロトモグラフィによる研究

Gu L, Wei X, Ling J, Huang X.

　未処置のイスムスは、歯内療法の失敗原因の1つとなる可能性がある。われわれはエックス線CT(マイクロトモグラフィ)スキャンを用いて下顎第一大臼歯近心根のイスムスの解剖学的特徴を検索した。36本の下顎第一大臼歯抜去歯が中国人から採取され、そして年齢別に以下の3群に分類された。Group A：20－39歳、Gropu B：40－59歳、Group C：60歳以上。各歯はスキャンされ、画像再構築をされた後、イスムスの出現率およびイスムスのタイプが記録された。イスムスが観察されたCT画像の割合は、Group A：50％、Group B：41％、そしてGroup C：24％であった。カイ二乗検定において、イスムスの出現率と年齢との間に有意な相関が認められた(P＜0.001)。部分的イスムスと完全イスムスの出現比は、Group A(5.9：1)やGroup B(7.0：1)よりも、Group C(17.1：1)が有意に高かった(P＜0.001)。イスムスの形状や位置を理解することにより、さらに効果的なエンドドンティック・マイクロサージェリーが保証されるであろう。

(J Endod 2009；35(3)：353-356.)

Untreated isthmuses can be a cause of endodontic treatment failure. We investigated the anatomic features of the isthmus in the mesial root of mandibular first molars using microcomputed tomography scans. Thirty-six extracted mandibular first molars were collected from the Chinese population and divided into three age groups as follows: 20 to 39 years (group A), 40 to 59 years (group B), and >or=60 years (group C). Each tooth was scanned and reconstructed, and then the prevalence and type of isthmus were recorded. The percentage of sections showing isthmuses for groups A, B, and C were 50%, 41%, and 24%, respectively. The chi-square test indicated a significant correlation of the distribution of isthmuses with age (p<0.001). The ratio of partial isthmus to complete isthmus for group C (17.1:1) was significantly higher than group A (5.9:1) and group B (7.0:1) (p<0.001).By understanding the configuration and location of isthmus, a more efficient endodontic microsurgery can be guaranteed.

Endodontic microsurgery

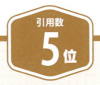

Five-year longitudinal assessment of the prognosis of apical microsurgery.

根尖部マイクロサージェリーの予後に関する5年の長期評価

von Arx T, Jensen SS, Hänni S, Friedman S.

緒言：根尖外科手術は、根尖性歯周炎を有する歯に対する重要な治療選択オプションのひとつである。他の治療法と根尖外科手術を比較するためには、その長期予後の知識が必要である。本研究は根尖外科手術5年予後を評価するとともに、われわれの前報において用いた根尖外科手術1年予後症例との予測変数を評価した。

方法：逆根管充填材 SuperEBA（Staident International、Staines、UK）、MTA（ProRoot MTA；Dentsply Tulsa Dental Specialties、Tulsa、OK）、あるいはコンポジットレジン Retroplast（Retroplast Trading、Rorvig、Denmark）のいずれかを用いた逆根管充填をともなった根尖切除術が、同一の術式を用いて行われた。根尖切除術1年予後を評価した被験者（n＝191）は、臨床的評価とエックス線写真的評価のために術後5年経過して招致された。3名の試験官による独自の盲検的評価に基づいて、「治癒あるいは非治癒」の2値で治療結果を判定し、そしてロジスティック回帰分析により患者、歯、治療に関する変数と治療結果とが関連づけて算出された。

結果：根尖切除術5年経過後において、191本中9歯が追跡不能、そして12歯が抜歯されたため、残りの170歯を本研究の検索対象とした（リコール率87.6％）。根尖切除術1年経過後では治癒率は83.8％であったが、5年経過後では75.9％（170本中129歯）が治癒と判定され、そして85.3％は無症状であった。（本研究の結果から、）2つの重要な予後因子が明らかとなった。1つ目はセメント-エナメル境からの近遠心的な歯槽骨レベルが3mm以内（治癒率78.2％）であるか3mmよりも大きい（治癒率52.9％）のかということ（オッズ比5.10、信頼区間1.67-16.21；P＜0.02）。2つ目はProRoot MTA（治癒率86.4％）あるいはSuperEBA（治癒率67.3％）のどちらの逆根管充填材を用いたかということであった（オッズ比7.65、信頼区間2.60-25.27；P＜0.004）。

結論：本研究は、根尖部マイクロサージェリー後5年経過時の治癒成績は術後1年と比べて8％低くなることを示唆していた。また、患歯の隣接面の歯槽骨レベルと使用される逆根管充填材の種類によって、術後経過は有意な影響を受けることが示唆された。

（J Endod 2012；38(5)：570-579.）

INTRODUCTION: Apical surgery is an important treatment option for teeth with post-treatment apical periodontitis. Knowledge of the long-term prognosis is necessary when weighing apical surgery against alternative treatments. This study assessed the 5-year outcome of apical surgery and its predictors in a cohort for which the 1-year outcome was previously reported.
METHODS: Apical microsurgery procedures were uniformly performed using SuperEBA (Staident International, Staines, UK) or mineral trioxide aggregate (MTA) (ProRoot MTA; Dentsply Tulsa Dental Specialties, Tulsa, OK)root-end fillings or alternatively Retroplast capping (Retroplast Trading, Rorvig, Denmark). Subjects examined at 1 year (n=191) were invited for the 5-year clinical and radiographic examination. Based on blinded, independent assessment by 3 calibrated examiners, the dichotomous outcome (healed or nonhealed) was determined and associated with patient-, tooth-, and treatment-related variables using logistic regression.
RESULTS: At the 5-year follow-up, 9 of 191 teeth were unavailable, 12 of 191 teeth were extracted, and 170 of 191 teeth were examined (87.6% recall rate). A total of 129 of 170 teeth were healed (75.9%) compared with 83.8% at 1 year, and 85.3% were asymptomatic. Two significant outcome predictors were identified: the mesial-distal bone level at ≦3 mm versus >3 mm from the cementoenamel junction (78.2% vs. 52.9% healed, respectively; odds ratio=5.10; confidence interval, 1.67-16.21; P<.02) and root-end fillings with ProRoot MTA versus SuperEBA (86.4% vs. 67.3% healed, respectively; odds ratio=7.65; confidence interval, 2.60-25.27; P<.004).
CONCLUSIONS: This study suggested that the 5-year prognosis after apical microsurgery was 8% poorer than assessed at 1 year. It also suggested that the prognosis was significantly impacted by the interproximal bone levels at the treated tooth and by the type of root-end filling material used.

エンドのための重要20キーワード

Endodontic treatment outcomes
歯内療法の治療成績

　歯内療法は全体としては、およそ90%の成功率を示すことが多数の論文において報告されているが、根尖部エックス線透過像の認められる再根管治療症例においては、成功率はおよそ60%程度に減少してしまう。そこで、本稿では、歯内療法の予後成績についての要因を検索した論文を主に紹介していく。

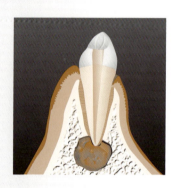

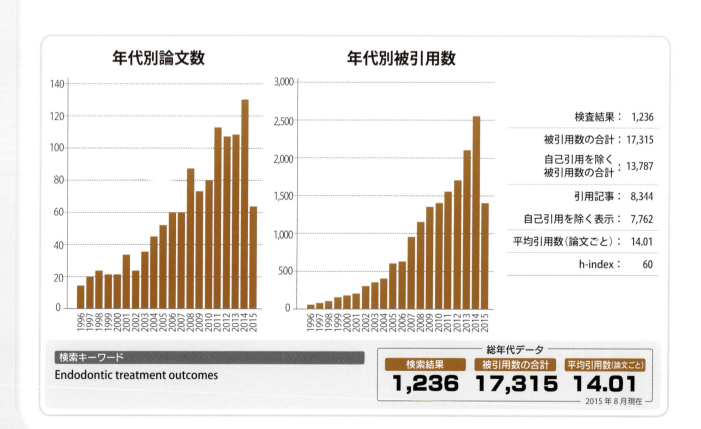

検索キーワード: Endodontic treatment outcomes

検査結果: 1,236
被引用数の合計: 17,315
自己引用を除く被引用数の合計: 13,787
引用記事: 8,344
自己引用を除く表示: 7,762
平均引用数(論文ごと): 14.01
h-index: 60

総年代データ
検索結果 1,236 / 被引用数の合計 17,315 / 平均引用数(論文ごと) 14.01
2015年8月現在

15 Endodontic treatment outcomes

トムソン・ロイターが選んだベスト12論文

順位	タイトル・和訳	2011年	2012年	2013年	2014年	合計引用数
引用数1位	Sundqvist G, Figdor D, Persson S, Sjögren U. Microbiologic analysis of teeth with failed endodontic treatment and the outcome of conservative re-treatment. Oral Surg Oral Med Oral Pathol Oral Radiol Endod 1998；85（1）：86-93. 歯内療法を失敗した歯の細菌学的解析と再保存治療の治療成績　**本項に和訳あり**	31	38	39	36	549
引用数2位	Sjogren U, Hagglund B, Sundqvist G, Wing K. Factors affecting the long-term results of endodontic treatment. J Endod 1990；16(10)：498-504. 根管治療の長期予後成績に影響する因子　**本項に和訳あり**	33	37	32	35	543
引用数3位	Sjögren U, Figdor D, Persson S, Sundqvist G. Influence of infection at the time of root filling on the outcome of endodontic treatment of teeth with apical periodontitis. Int Endod J 1997；30（5）：297-306. 根尖性歯周炎を有する歯の歯内療法の治療成績に対する根管充填時の感染の影響　**本項に和訳あり**	32	24	32	25	414
引用数4位	Peters OA. Current challenges and concepts in the preparation of root canal systems：a review. J Endod 2004；30（8）：559-567. 根管系の形成における現在の挑戦とコンセプト：総説論文　**本項に和訳あり**	28	29	30	41	276
引用数5位	Goodacre CJ, Bernal G, Rungcharassaeng K, Kan JY. Clinical complications in fixed prosthodontics. J Prosthet Dent 2003；90（1）：31-41. 固定性補綴物における臨床の合併症	20	14	29	25	187
引用数6位	Sundqvist G. Ecology of the root canal flora. J Endod 1992；18（9）：427-430. 根管の細菌叢の生態学	17	11	7	9	179
引用数7位	Tronstad L, Asbjørnsen K, Døving L, Pedersen I, Eriksen HM. Influence of coronal restorations on the periapical health of endodontically treated teeth. Endod Dent Traumatol 2000；16（5）：218-221. 歯内治療歯の根尖部の健全性に対する歯冠修復物の影響	14	8	10	10	143

エンドのための重要20キーワード（関連性の高い論文和訳）

トムソン・ロイターが選んだベスト12論文

	タイトル・和訳	2011年	2012年	2013年	2014年	合計引用数
引用数 8位	Siqueira JF Jr, Rôças IN. Clinical implications and microbiology of bacterial persistence after treatment procedures. J Endod 2008；34(11)：1291-1301. 治療後の細菌の持続感染の臨床的意味と微生物学	19	19	31	30	143
引用数 9位	Salehrabi R, Rotstein I. Endodontic treatment outcomes in a large patient population in the USA：an epidemiological study. J Endod 2004；30(12)：846-850. 米国の多数の患者人口における歯内治療の成功：疫学的研究	16	11	12	17	135
引用数 10位	Siqueira JF Jr. Endodontic infections：concepts, paradigms, and perspectives. Oral Surg Oral Med Oral Pathol Oral Radiol Endod 2002；94(3)：281-293. 歯内療法の感染：概念、凡例、および展望	8	6	14	11	118
引用数 11位	Mannocci F, Bertelli E, Sherriff M, Watson TF, Ford TR. Three-year clinical comparison of survival of endodontically treated teeth restored with either full cast coverage or with direct composite restoration. J Prosthet Dent 2002；88(3)：297-301. 全部鋳造冠あるいはコンポジットレジンの直接法による充填のいずれかで処置された歯内処置歯の3年生存率の臨床的比較	7	9	10	8	104
引用数 12位	Buckley M, Spångberg LS. The prevalence and technical quality of endodontic treatment in an American subpopulation. Oral Surg Oral Med Oral Pathol Oral Radiol Endod 1995；79(1)：92-100. 米国人の亜集団における歯内治療の有病率と治療技術の質	7	7	4	3	100

Endodontic treatment outcomes

Microbiologic analysis of teeth with failed endodontic treatment and the outcome of conservative re-treatment.

歯内療法を失敗した歯の細菌学的解析と再保存治療の治療成績

Sundqvist G, Figdor D, Persson S, Sjögren U.

目的：本研究の目的は歯内療法を失敗した歯にどのような細菌叢が存在するのかを確定し、保存的な再治療の成績を確かめることであった。

研究のデザイン：持続的な根尖病変を有する根管充填歯54本を、再根管治療のために選んだ。根管充填材を除去した後、根管から先進的な細菌学的技術手法により標本抽出を行った。その歯を再治療した後、5年に至るまで経過観察した。

結果：細菌叢は、主にグラム陽性菌が主体となった単一種で構成されていた。もっともよく回収された菌は、*Enterococcus faecalis* 系の細菌であった。全体の再治療の成功率は74％であった。

結論：失敗した歯内療法後の根管内の細菌叢は、未処置の細菌叢とは明らかに異なっていた。根管充填時の感染や根尖病変の大きさは、予後に悪影響を与える要因であった。歯内療法を失敗した歯の3/4は再治療に成功した。

（Oral Surg Oral Med Oral Pathol Oral Radiol Endod 1998；85(1)：86-93.）

AIM: The purposes of this study were to determine what microbial flora were present in teeth after failed root canal therapy and to establish the outcome of conservative re-treatment.
STUDY DESIGN: Fifty-four root-filled teeth with persisting periapical lesions were selected for re-treatment. After removal of the root filling, canals were sampled by means of advanced microbiologic techniques. The teeth were then re-treated and followed for up to 5 years.
RESULTS: The microbial flora was mainly single species of predominantly gram-positive organisms. The isolates most commonly recovered were bacteria of the species *Enterococcus faecalis*. The overall success rate of re-treatment was 74%.
CONCLUSIONS: The microbial flora in canals after failed endodontic therapy differed markedly from the flora in untreated teeth. Infection at the time of root filling and size of the periapical lesion were factors that had a negative influence on the prognosis. Three of four endodontic failures were successfully managed by re-treatment.

Factors affecting the long-term results of endodontic treatment.

根管治療の長期予後成績に影響する因子

Sjogren U, Hagglund B, Sundqvist G, Wing K.

　根管治療の成績に影響する可能性のある種々の要因を356名の患者の治療後8年間から10年間にわたり評価した。治療の結果は術前の歯髄と根尖部組織の状態に直接依存していた。生活歯髄あるいは根尖部透過像のない失活歯髄の症例の成功率は96％以上であり、一方、歯髄壊死し、根尖部透過像のある症例の86％だけに根尖部の治癒を認めた。根管の全長を根管形成可能であったかどうかということと、根管充填の到達度が、治療の成功に有意な影響を与えた。根尖病変を有した根管充填歯において、62％だけが術後の治癒が認められた。術前に根尖病変を有するそれぞれの症例において、臨床およびエックス線所見からの予見される治療の予後成績は、低いことがわかった。こうしたことから、測定や識別不能な要素も歯内療法の治療成績に重要であるかもしれない。

（J Endod 1990；16(10)：498-504.）

The influence of various factors that may affect the outcome of root canal therapy was evaluated in 356 patients 8 to 10 yr after the treatment. The results of treatment were directly dependent on the preoperative status of the pulp and periapical tissues. The rate of success for cases with vital or nonvital pulps but having no periapical radiolucency exceeded 96%, whereas only 86% of the cases with pulp necrosis and periapical radiolucency showed apical healing. The possibility of instrumenting the root canal to its full length and the level of root filling significantly affected the outcome of treatment. Of all of the periapical lesions present on previously root-filled teeth, only 62% healed after retreatment. The predictability from clinical and radiographic signs of the treatment-outcome in individual cases with preoperative periapical lesions cases was found to be low. Thus, factors which were not measured or identified may be critical to the outcome of endodontic treatment.

15 Endodontic treatment outcomes

Influence of infection at the time of root filling on the outcome of endodontic treatment of teeth with apical periodontitis.

根尖性歯周炎を有する歯の歯内療法の治療成績に対する根管充填時の感染の影響

Sjögren U, Figdor D, Persson S, Sundqvist G.

本研究は1回治療で根管清掃・充填された根管を有した歯の経過観察から歯内治療の予後に対する感染の役割を検索した。根尖性歯周炎の認められる単根歯55歯の根管に、徹底した根管形成と次亜塩素酸ナトリウムによる根管洗浄を行った。先進の嫌気性細菌学的技術を用いて根管形成後の細菌サンプルを採取後、その歯を同一治療時間内に根管充填した。すべての歯において術前の感染が認められた。根管形成後、少数の細菌が、55根管中22根管で検出された。根尖部における治癒は5年間経過観察された。根尖部の完全な治癒は、陰性培養であった症例の94％で起きていた。根管充填前に陽性であったサンプルでは、治療の成功率は、統計学的な有意差が認められ、ほんの68％であった。これらの失敗症例をさらに検索すると、それぞれの症例において*Actinomyces*種の存在が明らかとなり、失敗症例には関係するその他の細菌種は認められなかった。これらの所見は、根管充填前に根管系から細菌を完全に排除する重要性を強く示唆するものである。治療間における抗菌剤の根管貼薬のサポートなしに根管からすべての感染を根絶できないことから、この目的は1回治療では確実に達成することはできないと考えられる。

（Int Endod J 1997；30（5）：297-306.）

This study investigated the role of infection on the prognosis of endodontic therapy by following-up teeth that had had their canals cleaned and obturated during a single appointment. The root canals of 55 single-rooted teeth with apical periodontitis were thoroughly instrumented and irrigated with sodium hypochlorite solution. Using advanced anaerobic bacteriological techniques, post-instrumentation samples were taken and the teeth were then root-filled during the same appointment. All teeth were initially infected; after instrumentation low numbers of bacteria were detected in 22 of 55 root canals. Periapical healing was followed-up for 5 years. Complete periapical healing occurred in 94% of cases that yielded a negative culture. Where the samples were positive prior to root filling, the success rate of treatment was just 68%-a statistically significant difference. Further investigation of three failures revealed the presence of *Actinomyces species* in each case; no other specific bacteria were implicated in failure cases. These findings emphasize the importance of completely eliminating bacteria from the root canal system before obturation. This objective cannot be reliably achieved in a one-visit treatment because it is not possible to eradicate all infection from the root canal without the support of an inter-appointment antimicrobial dressing.

Current challenges and concepts in the preparation of root canal systems : a review.

根管系の形成における現在の挑戦とコンセプト：総説論文

Peters OA.

　Ni-Ti製ロータリーファイルは歯内療法における重要な周辺器具である。本総説では、これらのファイルを用いた根管形成の治療成績に影響する因子である術前における根管の解剖学的形態やファイル先端のデザインの明確化を試みる。重要度のより少ない因子として、ほかに、術者の経験、回転スピード、および特別なファイルシーケンスなどが挙げられる。さまざまな作業長の決定法および理想的な根尖部の拡大号数の決定法は、臨床結果と相関している。根管の解剖学的形態はつねに存在する1つの危険因子であるが、Ni-Ti製ロータリーファイルを用いた根管形成では、治療成績をもっとも予見可能である。現時点での研究報告は、より大きく根尖部の拡大形成を行うと、さらに良好な治療成績となることを示唆している。Ni-Ti製ロータリーファイルは、破折の危険性を最小限にするために臨床前に練習期間を設ける必要があり、そして症例に応じて作業長と根尖部の拡大号数を決定すべきである。*in vitro*における研究結果は優れたものであるが、Ni-Ti製ファイルを用いたときの治療成績を評価するためには、無作為に臨床試験を行うことも必要である。

（J Endod 2004；30（8）：559-567.）

> Nickel-titanium rotary instruments are important adjuncts in endodontic therapy. This review attempts to identify factors that influence shaping outcomes with these files, such as preoperative root-canal anatomy and instrument tip design. Other, less significant factors include operator experience, rotational speed, and specific instrument sequence. Implications of various working length definitions and desired apical widths are correlated with clinical results. Despite the existence of one ever-present risk factor, dental anatomy, shaping outcomes with nickel-titanium rotary instruments are mostly predictable. Current evidence indicates that wider apical preparations are feasible. Nickel-titanium rotary instruments require a preclinical training period to minimize separation risks and should be used to case-related working lengths and apical widths. However, and despite superior *in vitro* results, randomized, clinical trials are required to evaluate outcomes when using nickel-titanium instruments.

エンドのための重要20キーワード

16 Mineral trioxide aggregate
MTA

MTAは根管系を封鎖するために開発された材料であり、主原料はケイ酸三カルシウム（tricalcium silicate：Ca_3SiO_5）、アルミン酸三カルシウム（tricalcium aluminate：$Ca_3Al_2O_6$）、酸化三カルシウム、酸化ケイ酸塩である。MTAは親水性の粉末で、水と練和することでコロイド状のゲルとなる。硬化時間は4時間以内とされ、アマルガムと同様の硬さを有しているとされている。MTAの特徴として、比較的良好な封鎖性、高いpHによる抗菌性、生体親和性、および硬組織形成誘導能を有することなどが挙げられるが、操作性はあまり優れているとはいえず、練和の際の混水比にも注意が必要である。

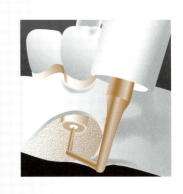

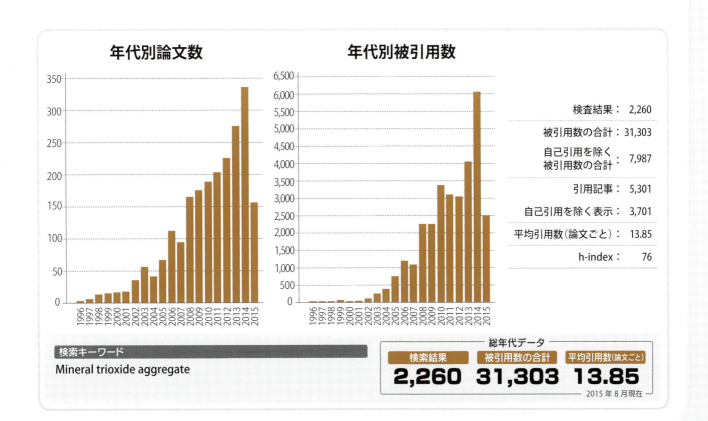

検査結果：	2,260
被引用数の合計：	31,303
自己引用を除く被引用数の合計：	7,987
引用記事：	5,301
自己引用を除く表示：	3,701
平均引用数（論文ごと）：	13.85
h-index：	76

検索キーワード
Mineral trioxide aggregate

総年代データ
検索結果	被引用数の合計	平均引用数（論文ごと）
2,260	31,303	13.85

2015年8月現在

トムソン・ロイターが選んだベスト12論文

	タイトル・和訳	2011年	2012年	2013年	2014年	合計引用数
引用数 1位	Torabinejad M, Hong CU, McDonald F, Pitt Ford TR. Physical and chemical properties of a new root-end filling material. J Endod 1995；21（7）：349-353. ある新しい逆根管充填材の物性および化学的性質 **本項に和訳あり**	37	38	38	52	474
引用数 2位	Torabinejad M, Chivian N. Clinical applications of mineral trioxide aggregate. J Endod 1999；25（3）：197-205. Mineral trioxide aggregate の臨床応用 **本項に和訳あり**	36	31	31	42	406
引用数 3位	Torabinejad M, Watson TF, Pitt Ford TR. Sealing ability of a mineral trioxide aggregate when used as a root end filling material. J Endod 1993；19(12)：591-595. 逆根管充填材として用いたときの mineral trioxide aggregate の封鎖性	30	31	22	40	393
引用数 4位	Lee SJ, Monsef M, Torabinejad M. Sealing ability of a mineral trioxide aggregate for repair of lateral root perforations. J Endod 1993；19(11)：541-544. 根管部側方のパーフォレーションリペアに対する mineral trioxide aggregate の封鎖性 **本項に和訳あり**	28	21	21	30	311
引用数 5位	Sarkar NK, Caicedo R, Ritwik P, Moiseyeva R, Kawashima I. Physico-chemical basis of the biologic properties of mineral trioxide aggregate. J Endod 2005；31（2）：97-100. mineral trioxide aggregate の生物学的性質の物理化学的な原理	25	26	28	40	229
引用数 6位	Torabinejad M, Pitt Ford TR, McKendry DJ, Abedi HR, Miller DA, Kariyawasam SP. Histologic assessment of mineral trioxide aggregate as a root-end filling in monkeys. J Endod 1997；23（4）：225-228. サルに逆根管充填したときの mineral trioxide aggregate の組織学的評価	21	8	8	10	215
引用数 7位	Koh ET, McDonald F, Pitt Ford TR, Torabinejad M. Cellular response to Mineral Trioxide Aggregate. J Endod 1998；24（8）：543-547. mineral trioxide aggregate への細胞応答	16	8	13	19	214

16 Mineral trioxide aggregate

トムソン・ロイターが選んだベスト12論文

順位	タイトル・和訳	2011年	2012年	2013年	2014年	合計引用数
引用数 8位	Torabinejad M, Hong CU, Lee SJ, Monsef M, Pitt Ford TR. Investigation of mineral trioxide aggregate for root-end filling in dogs. J Endod 1995；21(12)：603-608. イヌの逆根管充填に用いた mineral trioxide aggregate の研究 **本項に和訳あり**	16	10	5	13	206
引用数 9位	Banchs F, Trope M. Revascularization of immature permanent teeth with apical periodontitis：new treatment protocol? J Endod 2004；30(4)：196-200. 根尖性歯周炎をともなう幼若永久歯のリバスクラリセーション：新しい治療のプロトコール？ **チャプター18に和訳あり**	23	23	43	44	206
引用数 10位	Torabinejad M, Rastegar AF, Kettering JD, Pitt Ford TR. Bacterial leakage of mineral trioxide aggregate as a root-end filling material. J Endod 1995；21(3)：109-112. 逆根管充填材としての mineral trioxide aggregate の細菌漏洩	14	10	5	8	190
引用数 11位	Parirokh M, Torabinejad M. Mineral trioxide aggregate：a comprehensive literature review — Part Ⅰ：chemical, physical, and antibacterial properties. J Endod 2010；36(1)：16-27. Mineral trioxide aggregate：広範な文献レビュー—パート１：化学的、物理的、および抗菌的性質	28	36	44	51	184
引用数 12位	Torabinejad M, Higa RK, McKendry DJ, Pitt Ford TR. Dye leakage of four root end filling materials：effects of blood contamination. J Endod 1994；20(4)：159-163. ４種の逆根管充填材の色素漏洩：血液汚染の影響	13	8	8	10	180

Physical and chemical properties of a new root-end filling material.

ある新しい逆根管充填材の物性および化学的性質

Torabinejad M, Hong CU, McDonald F, Pitt Ford TR.

　本研究はMineral Trioxide Aggregate (MTA) の化学組成、pH、およびエックス線不透過性を測定することであり、そしてまた、この材料の硬化時間、圧縮強さ、および溶解性を、アマルガム、Super-EBA セメント、および IRM (Intermediate Restorative Material) セメントと比較することであった。走査型電子顕微鏡と一緒にエネルギー分散型エックス線分析装置を MTA の化学組成の測定に用い、そして、MTA の pH 値を、温度補正電極を備えた pH メーターで評価した。MTA のエックス線不透過性は ISO (International Organization for Standardization) により定められた方法で測定した。これらの材料の硬化時間と圧縮強さは BSI (British Standards Institution) により推奨された方法により測定した。材料の溶解度は ADA (American Dental Association) 指針を改良して評価した。研究結果は MTA 中の主たる分子はカルシウムとリン酸イオンであることを示していた。さらに MTA は最初 pH10.2 であったが、練和 3 時間経過後には pH12.5 に上昇した。MTA は、Super-EBA セメントや IRM セメントよりもエックス線不透過性が高かった。アマルガムの硬化時間は 4 分ともっとも短く、そして、MTA は 2 時間45分ともっとも長かった。24時間経過時、MTA は 40MPa ともっとも低い圧縮強さであったが、21日経過時には 67MPa ともっとも大きな圧縮強さであった。最後に、IRM セメントを除いた材料のいずれもが、本実験条件下では溶解性を示さなかった。

(J Endod 1995；21(7)：349-353.)

This study determined the chemical composition, pH, and radiopacity of mineral trioxide aggregate (MTA), and also compared the setting time, compressive strength, and solubility of this material with those of amalgam, Super-EBA, and Intermediate Restorative Material (IRM). X-ray energy dispersive spectrometer in conjunction with the scanning electron microscope were used to determine the composition of MTA, and the pH value of MTA was assessed with a pH meter using a temperature-compensated electrode. The radiopacity of MTA was determined according to the method described by the International Organization for Standardization. The setting time and compressive strength of these materials were determined according to methods recommended by the British Standards Institution. The degree of solubility of the materials was assessed according to modified American Dental Association specifications. The results showed that the main molecules present in MTA are calcium and phosphorous ions. In addition, MTA has a pH of 10.2 initially, which rises to 12.5 three hours after mixing. MTA is more radiopaque than Super-EBA and IRM. Amalgam had the shortest setting time (4 min) and MTA the longest (2 h 45 min). At 24 h MTA had the lowest compressive strength (40 MPa) among the materials, but it increased after 21 days to 67 MPa. Finally, except for IRM, none of the materials tested showed any solubility under the conditions of this study.

Clinical applications of mineral trioxide aggregate.

Mineral trioxide aggregate の臨床応用

Torabinejad M, Chivian N.

　実験材料のひとつである Mineral Trioxide Aggregate(MTA)は、現行の歯内療法で用いられている材料に取って代わる可能性のある修復材として近年研究されている。MTA は微小漏洩を防ぐこと、生体親和性のあること、そしてその材料が歯髄や根尖歯周組織に接して置かれた場合にもとの組織の再生を誘導することを、いくつかの in vitro と in vivo における研究は示している。本論文では、逆根管充填材として使用した場合について、さらに可逆性歯髄炎の直接覆髄、アペキシフィケーション、および非外科的あるいは外科的な根管部のパーフォレーションリペアについて MTA を用いた臨床処置について説明する。

(J Endod 1999;25(3):197-205.)

An experimental material, mineral trioxide aggregate (MTA), has recently been investigated as a potential alternative restorative material to the presently used materials in endodontics. Several *in vitro* and *in vivo* studies have shown that MTA prevents microleakage, is biocompatible, and promotes regeneration of the original tissues when it is placed in contact with the dental pulp or periradicular tissues. This article describes the clinical procedures for application of MTA in capping of pulps with reversible pulpitis, apexification, repair of root perforations nonsurgically and surgically, as well as its use as a root-end filling material.

Sealing ability of a mineral trioxide aggregate for repair of lateral root perforations.

根管部側方のパーフォレーションリペアに対する mineral trioxide aggregate の封鎖性

Lee SJ, Monsef M, Torabinejad M.

　アマルガム、IRM セメント、および MTA を、実験的に生じさせた歯根のパーフォレーションリペアについて試験した。50歯の正常下顎および上顎抜去歯が本研究に用いられた。パーフォレーションを、それぞれの歯の歯軸に対して約45°の角度で近心根表面に形成した。歯は、それから口腔内の状態を模擬するために生理食塩水に浸した吸水性スポンジ(Oasis)中に置かれた。パーフォレーション部に修復材料を充填した後、歯はその吸水性スポンジ中で、4週間保管された。その後、48時間メチレンブルーでパーフォレーション部を染色、薄切した後、解剖顕微鏡下において観察した。結果は、MTA は IRM セメントやアマルガムよりも有意に漏洩が少ないことを示していた。また、MTA は過剰充填が最小となる傾向を示し、一方、IRM セメントは充填不足が最小となる傾向を示した。

（J Endod 1993；19(11)：541-544.）

Amalgam, IRM, and a mineral trioxide aggregate were tested for repair of experimentally created root perforations. Fifty sound, extracted mandibular and maxillary molars were used in this study. A perforation was created on the mesial root surface at about a 45-degree angle to the long axis of each tooth. The tooth was then placed into a saline-soaked"Oasis"to simulate a clinical condition. After placing the repair materials into the perforations, the teeth were kept for 4 wk in the Oasis model. The perforation sites were then stained with methylene blue for 48 h, sectioned, and examined under a dissecting microscope. The results showed that the mineral trioxide aggregate had significantly less leakage than IRM or amalgam ($p<0.05$). The mineral trioxide aggregate also showed the least overfilling tendency while IRM showed the least underfilling tendency.

Mineral trioxide aggregate

Investigation of mineral trioxide aggregate for root-end filling in dogs.

イヌの逆根管充填に用いた mineral trioxide aggregate の研究

Torabinejad M, Hong CU, Lee SJ, Monsef M, Pitt Ford TR.

　多数の化合物が逆根管充填材として用いられてきた。*in vitro* や骨内移植試験の結果に基づいて考えると、Mineral Trioxide Aggregate（MTA）は逆根管充填材としての可能性があるように思える。本研究の目的は、MTA とアマルガムに対するイヌ根尖周囲組織の反応を検索することであった。6 匹のビーグル犬における46 根の根尖周囲組織に根尖病変を生じさせた。半数の根管は、根管形成後、ガッタパーチャとシーラーで根管充填し、そして髄腔開拡窩洞は MTA で封鎖した。残りの半数の根管は、根管形成後、シーラーを使用せずにガッタパーチャのみで根管充填した。このグループの髄腔開拡窩洞は、封鎖せずに口腔内に開放したままにした。外科的歯根切除後、逆根管充填窩洞の半数はアマルガムで充填し、残りは MTA で充填した。イヌ根尖周囲組織の反応は、根尖外科手術後 2 週から 5 週および10 週から18 週の観察期間で、組織学的に評価した。統計学的解析の結果より、アマルガムと比較して、MTA は根尖部の炎症がより小さいこと、そして MTA に近接したより多くの線維皮膜を認めることが、明らかとなった。さらに、MTA 表層におけるセメント質の存在が散見された。本研究結果は、MTA が逆根管充填材料として有用であることを示している。

（J Endod 1995；21（12）：603-608.）

Numerous compounds have been used as root-end filling materials. Based on the results of *in vitro* and intraosseous implantation tests, mineral trioxide aggregate (MTA) seems to have potential as a root-end filling material. The purpose of this study was to examine the periradicular tissue response of dogs to MTA and amalgam. Lesions were developed in periradicular tissues of 46 roots in six beagle dogs. The canals on half of the roots were instrumented and obturated with gutta-percha and sealer, and their access cavities were sealed with MTA. The remaining root canals were instrumented and obturated with gutta-percha and sealer, and their access cavities were sealed with MTA. The remaining root canals were instrumented and obturated with gutta-percha without root canal sealer. The access cavities of the teeth in this group were left open to the oral cavity. After surgical resection of roots, half of the root-end cavities were filled with amalgam and the rest with MTA. The periradicular tissue response of the dogs was evaluated histologically 2 to 5 and 10 to 18 wk following periradicular surgery. Statistical analysis of the results showed less periradicular inflammation and more fibrous capsules adjacent to MTA, compared with amalgam. In addition, the presence of cementum on the surface of MTA was a frequent finding. The results show that MTA can be used as a root-end filling material.

エンドのための重要20キーワード

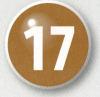

Cone-beam computed tomography
コーンビーム CT（CBCT）

近年 CT 装置は、医療技術の高度先進化にともない、歯科においても必要不可欠な存在となりつつある。コーンビーム CT（以下，CBCT と略）は、二次元検出器を用いているために、通常の CT 装置のような体軸方向への連続撮影が不要となっている。そのため、三次元像再構築に必要なエックス線投影像を短時間に低被曝で得られるという利点を有する。また、CBCT は、本来の立体的位置関係が再現でき、被写体の正確な立体的位置関係を三次元的に再現できるため、口内法エックス線撮影のような海綿骨などによる解剖学的なノイズを排除できる。

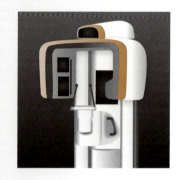

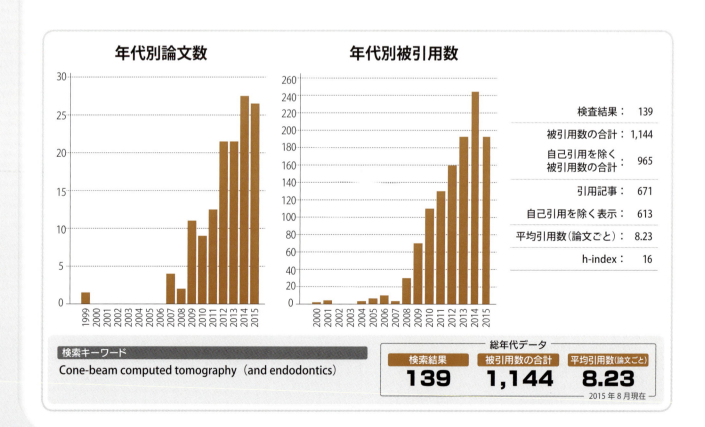

検索キーワード: Cone-beam computed tomography（and endodontics）

検査結果：	139
被引用数の合計：	1,144
自己引用を除く被引用数の合計：	965
引用記事：	671
自己引用を除く表示：	613
平均引用数（論文ごと）：	8.23
h-index：	16

総年代データ
- 検索結果：139
- 被引用数の合計：1,144
- 平均引用数（論文ごと）：8.23

2015 年 8 月現在

⑰ Cone-beam computed tomography

トムソン・ロイターが選んだベスト12論文

	タイトル・和訳	2011年	2012年	2013年	2014年	合計引用数
引用数 1位	Cotton TP, Geisler TM, Holden DT, Schwartz SA, Schindler WG. Endodontic applications of cone-beam volumetric tomography. J Endod 2007;33(9):1121-1132. コーンビーム断層撮影法(CBVT)の歯内療法への応用 **本項に和訳あり**	23	21	16	20	137
引用数 2位	Rhodes JS, Ford TR, Lynch JA, Liepins PJ, Curtis RV. Micro-computed tomography: a new tool for experimental endodontology. Int Endod J 1999;32(3):165-170. マイクロCT：実験的歯内療法学の新手段 **本項に和訳あり**	8	10	13	7	100
引用数 3位	Nair MK, Nair UP. Digital and advanced imaging in endodontics: a review. J Endod 2007;33(1):1-6. 歯内療法における先進的デジタル画像撮影：総説論文	12	16	8	8	100
引用数 4位	Patel S. New dimensions in endodontic imaging: Part 2. Cone beam computed tomography. Int Endod J 2009;42(6):463-475. 歯内療法の画像撮影における新次元：パート2. CBCT **本項に和訳あり**	24	22	15	19	99
引用数 5位	Patel S, Dawood A, Whaites E, Pitt Ford T. New dimensions in endodontic imaging: part 1. Conventional and alternative radiographic systems. Int Endod J 2009;42(6):447-462. 歯内療法の画像撮影における新次元：パート1．従来的および代替的エックス線撮影装置 **本項に和訳あり**	12	10	15	16	80
引用数 6位	Matherne RP, Angelopoulos C, Kulild JC, Tira D. Use of cone-beam computed tomography to identify root canal systems in vitro. J Endod 2008;34(1):87-89. In vitro において根管系を特定するためのCBCTの使用	10	12	15	12	79
引用数 7位	Patel S, Dawood A, Mannocci F, Wilson R, Pitt Ford T. Detection of periapical bone defects in human jaws using cone beam computed tomography and intraoral radiography. Int Endod J 2009;42(6):507-515. CBCTと口腔内エックス線撮影を用いたヒト顎における根尖部骨欠損の検出	11	15	8	11	57

129

トムソン・ロイターが選んだベスト**12**論文

	タイトル・和訳	2011年	2012年	2013年	2014年	合計引用数
引用数 **8位**	Tu MG, Huang HL, Hsue SS, Hsu JT, Chen SY, Jou MJ, Tsai CC. Detection of permanent three-rooted mandibular first molars by cone-beam computed tomography imaging in Taiwanese individuals. J Endod 2009；35（4）：503-507. CBCT画像撮影による台湾人の3根管性下顎第一大臼歯の発見	6	5	7	5	36
引用数 **9位**	Michetti J, Maret D, Mallet JP, Diemer F. Validation of cone beam computed tomography as a tool to explore root canal anatomy. J Endod 2010；36（7）：1187-1190. 根管解剖探査の手段として用いるCBCTの妥当性に対する検証	1	11	9	8	36
引用数 **10位**	Petersson A, Axelsson S, Davidson T, Frisk F, Hakeberg M, Kvist T, Norlund A, Mejàre I, Portenier I, Sandberg H, Tranaeus S, Bergenholtz G. Radiological diagnosis of periapical bone tissue lesions in endodontics：a systematic review. Int Endod J 2012；45（9）：783-801. 歯内療法における根尖部骨組織病変のエックス線診断	0	1	6	10	27
引用数 **11位**	Tsurumachi T, Honda K. A new cone beam computerized tomography system for use in endodontic surgery. Int Endod J 2007；40（3）：224-232. 外科的歯内療法用の新しいCBCT装置	4	6	1	1	23
引用数 **12位**	Tsai P, Torabinejad M, Rice D, Azevedo B. Accuracy of cone-beam computed tomography and periapical radiography in detecting small periapical lesions. J Endod 2012；38（7）：965-970. 小さい根尖病変の検出におけるCBCTと根尖部エックス線の精度	0	0	7	8	23

Cone-beam computed tomography

Endodontic applications of cone-beam volumetric tomography.

コーンビーム断層撮影法（CBVT）の歯内療法への応用

Cotton TP, Geisler TM, Holden DT, Schwartz SA, Schindler WG.

　関心のある部位を三次元で診査できることは、初心者のみならずベテラン臨床家の双方に同様に有益であろう。高解像度で小照射野のコーンビーム断層撮影法（CBVT）が歯科応用のために設計された。従来のCT画像の断層画像データと対照的に、CBVTは1度の撮影で円柱体積化したデータの取り込みをするため、従来の医科用CTと比べて有利な点を有する。これらの利点には、正確性、より高い解像度、操作時間の短縮、および放射線量の低減が含まれる。CBVTの歯内療法特有の応用は、このCBVT技術がより一般的になってきたものとして認識されている。CBVTは最新の歯内治療における重要な手段となる大きな可能性を有している。本論文の目的は、CBCT技術および医科のCTや従来法エックス線撮影と比べて有利な点を簡潔に論評し、歯内治療における現在および将来のCBCTの臨床応用を説明し、そして三次元データの取り込みと読影に属する医療の法律的側面に関する配慮について論じることである。

（J Endod 2007；33（9）：1121-1132.）

The ability to assess an area of interest in 3 dimensions might benefit both novice and experienced clinicians alike. High-resolution limited cone-beam volumetric tomography (CBVT) has been designed for dental applications. As opposed to sliced-image data of conventional computed tomography (CT) imaging, CBVT captures a cylindrical volume of data in one acquisition and thus offers distinct advantages over conventional medical CT. These advantages include increased accuracy, higher resolution, scan-time reduction, and dose reduction. Specific endodontic applications of CBVT are being identified as the technology becomes more prevalent. CBVT has great potential to become a valuable tool in the modern endodontic practice. The objectives of this article are to briefly review cone-beam technology and its advantages over medical CT and conventional radiography, to illustrate current and future clinical applications of cone-beam technology in endodontic practice, and to discuss medicolegal considerations pertaining to the acquisition and interpretation of 3-dimensional data.

Micro-computed tomography: a new tool for experimental endodontology.

マイクロCT：実験的歯内療法学の新手段

Rhodes JS, Ford TR, Lynch JA, Liepins PJ, Curtis RV.

目的：コーンビームジオメトリを用いたマイクロCTは、小さな標本構造の三次元画像を作成する方法のひとつである。試作マイクロCT装置が根管形成の定量化に用いることが可能かどうかを検索することを目的として、この試作マイクロCTを歯の画像処理化に適用した。

方法：未処置の歯冠と完全に完成した歯根を有する下顎第一大臼歯10歯を、マイクロCTを用いて0.081mmの解像度でスキャンした後、これから根管を断片化し、そして三次元レンダリング画像を構築した。マイクロCTの再現性は根管の形と大きさで確認した。アクセスキャビティを髄腔に形成後、クラウンダウン法を用いて連続したテーパー状の形成で根管拡大した。それぞれの歯は、根管形成の前後で比較するために再スキャンされた。その後、歯根と根管の面積のデジタルビデオ化測定のため、あらかじめ決めておいた5か所の水平位で歯根を薄切した。ビデオ画像は、0.025mmの解像度であった。物理的切断面のデジタルビデオ画像は、その歯のマイクロCT再構築画像と比較された。それぞれの部位における根管（内面）と歯根（外面）の総面積を、マイクロCTの再構築画像とデジタルビデオ画像の両方から算出して比較した。

結果：マイクロCT画像とデジタルビデオ画像の間には、内面と外面の面積のどちらに対しても、有意に高い相関性が認められた（r＝0.94）。歯の根管系を再現した三次元レンダリング画像は構築できた。根尖から7.5mmまでの根管の総体積を根管形成前後の9歯のレンダリング画像から算出した。根管形成で削除された象牙質量の平均は、もとの根管の体積の28%に相当する$3.725mm^3$であった。

結論：実験的歯内療法に対するマイクロCTの正確性が示された。

（Int Endod J 1999；32（3）：165-170.）

AIM: Micro-computed tomography (MCT) using conebeam geometry is a method of producing true 3D images of the structure of small samples. A prototype MCT unit was adapted for imaging teeth to examine whether it could be used to quantify the instrumentation of root canals.
METHODOLOGY: Ten mandibular first molar teeth that had intact crowns and fully formed roots were scanned using MCT at a resolution of 0.081mm and 3D-rendered images created; root canals were segmented from this. Reproducibility of MCT was verified for root canal shape and size. Access cavities were prepared into the pulp space and root canals enlarged to a continously tapering preparation using a crowndown technique. Each tooth was scanned again to allow comparison of pre- and post-instrumentation images. The roots were then sectioned at five predetermined horizontal levels for video-digitized measurement of dimensions of roots and root canals. The video images had a resolution of 0.025mm. Video-digitized images of the physical cut surfaces were compared with equivalent MCT reconstructed images. The total area of the root canals (internal) and root (external) at each level were calculated from both MCT reconstructions and video-digitized images, and compared.
RESULTS: There was a highly significant correlation between MCT and video images for both external and internal areas (r=0.94). Rendered 3D images were constructed to show the root canal systems of teeth. The total volumes of the apical 7.5mm of root canals were calculated from rendered images of nine teeth before and after instrumentation. The mean amount of dentine removed by instrumentation was $3.725mm^3$ which was 28% of the original canal volume.
CONCLUSIONS: Micro-computed tomography was shown to be accurate for experimental endodontology.

Cone-beam computed tomography

New dimensions in endodontic imaging：
Part 2. Cone beam computed tomography.

歯内療法の画像撮影における新次元：
パート2．CBCT

Patel S.

　CBCTは、従来のCTと比較して有意に低影響の放射線量により、歯とその周囲組織を含む顎顔面骨の正確な三次元情報を生成するために特別に設計されている。CBCTを用いると根尖病変は根尖部エックス線写真と比較してより速やかに検出できるであろうし、病変の実際の大きさ、性状、および根尖と骨吸収性病変の位置も評価することができる。歯根破折、根管の解剖学的形態、および歯の周囲の顎骨の構造的特徴も評価できるであろう。本論文の目的は、歯内療法における難症例の対応におけるCBCTの応用と限界について最新文献を論評することである。

（Int Endod J 2009；42（6）：463-475.）

Cone beam computed tomography (CBCT) has been specifically designed to produce undistorted three-dimensional information of the maxillofacial skeleton, including the teeth and their surrounding tissues with a significantly lower effective radiation dose compared with conventional computed tomography (CT). Periapical disease may be detected sooner using CBCT compared with periapical views and the true size, extent, nature and position of periapical and resorptive lesions can be assessed. Root fractures, root canal anatomy and the nature of the alveolar bone topography around teeth may be assessed. The aim of this paper is to review current literature on the applications and limitations of CBCT in the management of endodontic problems.

New dimensions in endodontic imaging: part 1. Conventional and alternative radiographic systems.

歯内療法の画像撮影における新次元：パート1．従来的および代替的エックス線撮影装置

Patel S, Dawood A, Whaites E, Pitt Ford T

　難症例の対応に従来のエックス線写真を用いると、撮影画像の二次元的な特性や、幾何学的な歪み、そして解剖学的なノイズのために限られた情報しか得られない。これらの要因は、しばしば重なって同時に発生する。本総説論文では根尖部エックス線写真の限界を評価し、従来のエックス線写真に加わるべき三次元画像診断法を明確にする。これらには、TACT（Tuned Aperture Computed Tomography）、MRI（Magnetic Resonance Imaging）、超音波、CT、およびCBCTが含まれる。これらの技術のうち、CBCTは従来のエックス線写真に関するいくつかの問題を解決するために効果的かつ安全であると思われる。

(Int Endod J 2009 ; 42 (6) : 447-462.)

> Conventional radiographs used for the management of endodontic problems yield limited information because of the two-dimensional nature of images produced, geometric distortion and anatomical noise. These factors often act in combination. This review paper assesses the limitations of periapical radiographs and seeks to clarify three-dimensional imaging techniques that have been suggested as adjuncts to conventional radiographs. These include tuned aperture computed tomography, magnetic resonance imaging, ultrasound, computed tomography and cone beam computed tomography (CBCT). Of these techniques, CBCT appears to be an effective and safe way to overcome some of the problems associated with conventional radiographs.

エンドのための重要20キーワード

18 *Pulp revascularization*
パルプ・リバスクラリゼーション

パルプ・リバスクラリゼーションの基本概念は、Nygaard-Østbyによる提案（Acta Odontol Scand 1961；19：324-353）に遡る。この報告の術式は、根尖性歯周炎を有する歯髄壊死を生じた歯の根管充填前にわざと根尖からファイルを突きだして血餅を作成する。そして、この血餅を足場として脈管系の新生を促し、新たな組織が再生することを期待するという手法であった。岩谷ら（本項に抄録の和訳あり）は、一部性に歯髄壊死を起こした幼若下顎第二小臼歯に対して行った歯内療法の症例をリバスクラリゼーション（revascularization）という言葉を用いて初めて報告した。以後、パルプ・リバスクラリゼーションに対する研究が、近年の再生医療技術の進歩と相まって、数多く報告されるようになる。

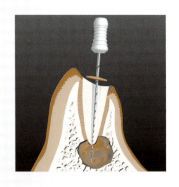

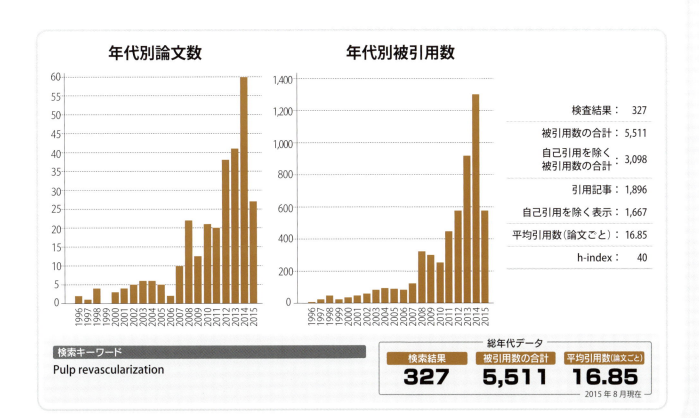

検索キーワード
Pulp revascularization

検査結果： 327
被引用数の合計： 5,511
自己引用を除く被引用数の合計： 3,098
引用記事： 1,896
自己引用を除く表示： 1,667
平均引用数（論文ごと）： 16.85
h-index： 40

総年代データ
検索結果 327
被引用数の合計 5,511
平均引用数（論文ごと） 16.85
2015年8月現在

トムソン・ロイターが選んだベスト12論文

	タイトル・和訳	2011年	2012年	2013年	2014年	合計引用数
引用数1位	Sonoyama W, Liu Y, Yamaza T, Tuan RS, Wang S, Shi S, Huang GT. Characterization of the apical papilla and its residing stem cells from human immature permanent teeth: a pilot study. J Endod 2008;34(2):166-171. ヒト幼若永久歯由来の歯乳頭と歯乳頭幹細胞の特性評価：予備実験 **本項に和訳あり**	46	46	58	60	277
引用数2位	Banchs F, Trope M. Revascularization of immature permanent teeth with apical periodontitis: new treatment protocol? J Endod 2004;30(4):196-200. 根尖性歯周炎をともなう幼若永久歯のリバスクラリゼーション：新しい治療のプロトコール？ **本項に和訳あり**	23	23	43	44	206
引用数3位	Murray PE, Garcia-Godoy F, Hargreaves KM. Regenerative endodontics: A review of current and a call for action. J Endod 2007;33(4):377-390. 再生歯内療法：現行法の総説と行動喚起 **本項に和訳あり**	23	15	23	24	148
引用数4位	Iwaya S, Ikawa M, Kubota M. Revascularization of an immature permanent tooth with apical periodontitis and sinus tract. Endod Dent Traumatol 2001;17(4):185-187. 根尖性歯周炎と瘻孔をともなう幼若永久歯のリバスクラリゼーション **本項に和訳あり**	17	11	32	30	145
引用数5位	Andreasen JO, Borum MK, Jacobsen HL, Andreasen FM. Replantation of 400 avulsed permanent incisors. 1. Diagnosis of healing complications. Endod Dent Traumatol 1995;11(2):51-58. 400本の脱落永久切歯の再植．1．治癒経過における合併症の診断 **本項に和訳あり**	9	9	16	5	132
引用数6位	Andreasen JO, Borum MK, Jacobsen HL, Andreasen FM. Replantation of 400 avulsed permanent incisors. 2. Factors related to pulpal healing. Endod Dent Traumatol 1995;11(2):59-68. 400本の脱落永久切歯の再植．2．歯髄治癒に関する原因	10	10	8	8	120

18 Pulp revascularization

トムソン・ロイターが選んだベスト12論文

	タイトル・和訳	2011年	2012年	2013年	2014年	合計引用数
引用数 7位	Kristerson L. Autotransplantation of human premolars. A clinical and radiographic study of 100 teeth. Int J Oral Surg 1985；14(2)：200-213. ヒト小臼歯の自家移植。臨床検査およびエックス線写真撮影を用いた100歯の研究	4	7	6	9	104
引用数 8位	Kling M, Cvek M, Mejare I. Rate and predictability of pulp revascularization in therapeutically reimplanted permanent incisors. Endod Dent Traumatol 1986；2(3)：83-89. 治療的に再移植された永久切歯におけるパルプ・リバスクラリゼーションの割合と予知性	5	9	12	10	104
引用数 9位	Chueh LH, Huang GT. Immature teeth with periradicular periodontitis or abscess undergoing apexogenesis：a paradigm shift. J Endod 2006；32(12)：1205-1213. 根尖性歯周炎あるいは根尖膿瘍を有したアペクソジェネシス中の幼若歯：パラダイムシフト	10	16	26	18	103
引用数 10位	Trope M. Clinical management of the avulsed tooth：present strategies and future directions. Dent Traumatol 2002；18(1)：1-11. 脱落歯の臨床管理：現在の戦略と今後の方向性	6	8	7	6	101
引用数 11位	Thibodeau B, Teixeira F, Yamauchi M, Caplan DJ, Trope M. Pulp revascularization of immature dog teeth with apical periodontitis. J Endod 2007；33(6)：680-689. 根尖性歯周炎を有した若齢犬の歯のパルプ・リバスクラリゼーション	13	9	20	26	100
引用数 12位	Skoglund A, Tronstad L, Wallenius K. A microangiographic study of vascular changes in replanted and autotransplanted teeth of young dogs. Oral Surg Oral Med Oral Pathol 1978；45(1)：17-28. 若齢犬の再植歯と自家移植歯の血管変化の微小血管造影法を用いた研究	2	6	3	6	93

Characterization of the apical papilla and its residing stem cells from human immature permanent teeth : a pilot study.

ヒト幼若永久歯由来の歯乳頭と歯乳頭幹細胞の特性評価：予備実験

Sonoyama W, Liu Y, Yamaza T, Tuan RS, Wang S, Shi S, Huang GT.

　間葉系幹細胞は永久歯の歯髄組織（歯髄幹細胞もしくはDPSCs）や乳歯（ヒト脱落乳歯幹細胞）から単離されてきた。われわれは、最近、歯乳頭幹細胞と呼ばれるヒト幼若永久歯の歯乳頭に存在する別種の間葉系幹細胞を発見した。ここでは、われわれはさらに、組織学的、免疫組織化学的、および免疫細胞蛍光分析を用いて、歯乳頭組織および歯乳頭幹細胞の幹細胞的特徴を特性解析した。歯乳頭は、歯髄と比較して細胞および血管要素が少ない点で歯髄と異なることをわれわれは発見した。器官培養において歯乳頭細胞は歯髄細胞よりも2から3倍多く増殖した。歯乳頭幹細胞と歯髄幹細胞は両方とも、骨髄由来間葉系幹細胞と同程度の骨形成/象牙質形成細胞への分化能があったが、一方、脂肪形成能では劣った。歯乳頭幹細胞の免疫表現型は、骨形成/象牙質形成と成長因子受容体の遺伝子プロファイルに関して歯髄幹細胞と類似している。培養歯乳頭幹細胞における二重染色実験は、STRO-1は骨シアロタンパク、オステオカルシンのような象牙質形成マーカーと、そして増殖因子FGFR1やTGFbetaRIと共発現することを示した。さらに、神経細胞培地の刺激により歯乳頭幹細胞はネスチンやニューロフィラメント-Mといった多様な神経性マーカーを発現する。歯乳頭幹細胞は歯髄幹細胞と類似しているが、歯髄能幹細胞/前駆細胞とは由来が異なるとわれわれは結論づけた。歯根の成長およびアペクソジェネシスにおける歯乳頭幹細胞との関連が考察される。

（J Endod 2008；34（2）：166-171.）

Mesenchymal stem cells (MSCs) have been isolated from the pulp tissue of permanent teeth (dental pulp stem cells or DPSCs) and deciduous teeth (stem cells from human exfoliated deciduous teeth). We recently discovered another type of MSCs in the apical papilla of human immature permanent teeth termed stem cells from the apical papilla (SCAP). Here, we further characterized the apical papilla tissue and stem cell properties of SCAP using histologic, immunohistochemical, and immunocytofluorescent analyses. We found that the apical papilla is distinctive to the pulp in terms of containing less cellular and vascular components than those in the pulp. Cells in the apical papilla proliferated 2- to 3-fold greater than those in the pulp in organ cultures. Both SCAP and DPSCs were as potent in osteo/dentinogenic differentiation as MSCs from bone marrows, whereas they were weaker in adipogenic potential. The immunophenotype of SCAP is similar to that of DPSCs on the osteo/dentinogenic and growth factor receptor gene profiles. Double-staining experiments showed that STRO-1 coexpressed with dentinogenic markers such as bone sialophosphoprotein, osteocalcinm, and growth factors FGFR1 and TGFbetaRI in cultured SCAP. Additionally, SCAP express a wide variety of neurogenic markers such as nestin and neurofilament M upon stimulation with a neurogenic medium. We conclude that SCAP are similar to DPSCs but a distinct source of potent dental stem/progenitor cells. Their implications in root development and apexogenesis are discussed.

Revascularization of immature permanent teeth with apical periodontitis : new treatment protocol ?

根尖性歯周炎をともなう幼若永久歯のリバスクラリゼーション：
新しい治療のプロトコール？

Banchs F, Trope M.

　根尖性歯周炎をともなう幼若永久歯にリバスクラリゼーションを起こすための新しい手法を提案する。根管に十分な洗浄と3種抗生剤による消毒を行う。この根管消毒が終了した後、セメント-エナメル境まで血餅を作成するため、根尖歯周組織を機械的に刺激して根管内へ出血させる。それから髄腔開拡部の二重仮封を行う。本症例においては、根管消毒、新生組織の増殖可能なマトリックス、そして効果的な歯冠部の封鎖の組み合わせにより、効果的なリバスクラリゼーションに必要な環境が作りだされたと考えられる。

（J Endod 2004 ; 30（4）: 196-200.）

A new technique is presented to revascularize immature permanent teeth with apical periodontitis. The canal is disinfected with copious irrigation and a combination of three antibiotics. After the disinfection protocol is complete, the apex is mechanically irritated to initiate bleeding into the canal to produce a blood clot to the level of the cemento-enamel junction. The double seal of the coronal access is then made. In this case, the combination of a disinfected canal, a matrix into which new tissue could gro, and an effective coronal seal appears to have produced the environment necessary for successful revascularization.

Regenerative endodontics：
A review of current and a call for action.

再生歯内療法：現行法の総説と行動喚起

Murray PE, Garcia-Godoy F, Hargreaves KM.

　根管治療により、毎年、何百万本もの歯が救われている。現行の治療法でも多くの症例が高い確率で成功となるが、本治療のあるべき姿は、歯を生き返らすために、病的歯髄あるいは壊死歯髄を除去し、健康な歯髄組織に置き換えることを目的とした再生学的なアプローチとなるであろう。研究者たちはこの目標に向けて研究を続けている。再生歯内療法とは、病的な歯髄、欠損した歯髄、そして外傷を被った歯髄にとって代わる組織を作成し、供給することである。本総説では、再生歯内療法の概要とその目標について提供し、再生歯内療法を実現可能な手法を説明する。これらの将来性があるアプローチには、リバスクラリゼーション、成体幹細胞治療、歯髄移植、スキャホールド移植、三次元的生細胞プリンティング、流動性スキャホールド、そして遺伝子治療が含まれる。これらの再生歯内療法の技術は、リバスクラリゼーションを目的とする根尖部拡大を行い、感染根管消毒や汚染物質の除去し、そして成体幹細胞、スキャホールドや成長因子を用いるようないくつかの治療技術の組み合わせも含まれる。これらの歯内再生組織療法の挑戦は現実的なものとはいえ、患者や研究者への歯内再生組織療法の潜在的利益は一様に革新的である。組織工学的な治療は、人工補綴物の外科的な装着の代わりに、生来の機能を回復する可能性を与えるため、仕様や費用における患者要求はとても大きい。ここで再生歯内療法の発展に必要な手法を論じた論文のあらましを紹介することで、われわれはこれらの治療が臨床応用へ発展するための行動喚起が促されることを望む。

（J Endod 2007；33（4）：377-390.）

Millions of teeth are saved each year by root canal therapy. Although current treatment modalities offer high levels of success for many conditions, an ideal form of therapy might consist of regenerative approaches in which diseased or necrotic pulp tissues are removed and replaced with healthy pulp tissue to revitalize teeth. Researchers are working toward this objective. Regenerative endodontics is the creation and delivery of tissues to replace diseased, missing, and traumatized pulp. This review provides an overview of regenerative endodontics and its goals, and describes possible techniques that will allow regenerative endodontics to become a reality. These potential approaches include root-canal revascularization, postnatal (adult) stem cell therapy, pulp implant, scaffold implant, three-dimensional cell printing, injectable scaffolds, and gene therapy. These regenerative endodontic techniques will possibly involve some combination of disinfection or debridement of infected root canal systems with apical enlargement to permit revascularization and use of adult stem cells, scaffolds, and growth factors. Although the challenges of introducing endodontic tissue engineering therapies are substantial, the potential benefits to patients and the profession are equally ground breaking. Patient demand is staggering both in scope and cost, because tissue engineering therapy offers the possibility of restoring natural function instead of surgical placement of an artificial prosthesis. By providing an overview of the methodological issues required to develop potential regenerative endodontic therapies. we hope to present a call for action to develop these therapies for clinical use.

Pulp revascularization

Revascularization of an immature permanent tooth with apical periodontitis and sinus tract.

根尖性歯周炎と瘻孔をともなう幼若永久歯の
リバスクラリゼーション

Iwaya S, Ikawa M, Kubota M.

13歳の患者の壊死して根尖病変を認める幼若下顎第二小臼歯が治療された。標準的な根管治療手順やアペキシフィケーションに代わるものとして、根管を空のままにし、抗生剤を根管貼薬した。エックス線写真による検査では、抗生剤貼薬終了から5か月後に根尖の閉鎖が開始することが明らかになった。根管壁の肥厚と根尖の閉鎖の完成が、抗生剤貼薬終了後30か月に確認されたことから、無菌的な根管腔内に新しい(young)永久歯歯髄の再生(revascularization)が生じている可能性が示唆された。

(Endod Dent Traumatol 2001;17(4):185-187.)

A necrotic immature mandibular second premolar with periapical involvement in a 13-year-old patient was treated. Instead of the standard root canal treatment protocol and apexification, antimicrobial agents were used in the canal, after which the canal was left empty. Radiographic examination showed the start of apical closure 5 months after the completion of the antimicrobial protocol. Thickening of the canal wall and complete apical closure was confirmed 30 months after the treatment, indicating the revascularization potential of a young permanent tooth pulp into a bacteria-free root canal space.

Replantation of 400 avulsed permanent incisors.
1. Diagnosis of healing complications.

400本の脱落永久切歯の再植．
1．治癒経過における合併症の診断

Andreasen JO, Borum MK, Jacobsen HL, Andreasen FM.

　1965年から1988年までの観察期間（平均観察期間＝5.1年）において、脱落後、再植を施された永久歯400本を有する患者322名を検索対象として、予測調査を行った。再植時の患者の年齢の範囲は5歳から52歳（平均＝13.7歳、中央値11.0歳）であった。損傷の程度と加療法に関する有効データを得るため、規格化した患者記録を全期間に適用した。経過観察期間中は、臨床診断、動揺度検査、規格化エックス線写真撮影の管理による歯髄と歯周の治癒経過の観察を行った。再植歯のうち32本（8％）は歯髄治癒を示した。根未完成歯であるため、歯髄のリバスクラリゼーションが予想された94歯のうちの34％に歯髄治癒が観察された。歯根膜治癒（i.e. 歯根外部吸収の所見がない）は96歯（24％）で観察された。歯肉の治癒は371歯（93％）で観察された。観察期間中に、119歯（30％）は抜歯された。再植時における歯根の状態が根完成歯のほうが、歯根完成歯よりもわずかに多くであるが歯の喪失が起きた。

（Endod Dent Traumatol 1995；11（2）：51-58．）

A material of 322 patients with 400 avulsed and replanted permanent teeth were followed prospectively in the period from 1965 to 1988 (mean observation period=5.1 yrs). The age of the patients at the time of replantation ranged from 5 to 52 yrs (mean=13.7 yrs and median=11.0 yrs). Standardized patient records were used through the entire period in order to obtain valid data concerning the extent of injury and treatment provided. At the follow-up period, pulpal and periodontal healing were monitored by clinical examination, mobility testing and standardized radiographic controls. Thirty-two of the replanted teeth (8%) showed pulpal healing. When related to teeth with incomplete root formation, where pulpal revascularization was anticipated (n=94) the frequency of pulpal healing was 34%. Periodontal ligament healing (i.e. with no evidence of external root resorption) was found in 96 teeth (24%). Gingival healing was found in 371 teeth (93%). During the observation period, 119 teeth (30%) were extracted. Tooth loss was slightly more frequent in teeth with incomplete root formation at the time of replantation than in teeth with completed root formation.

エンドのための重要20キーワード

19 Dental pulp tissue engineering

歯髄組織工学

　不可逆性歯髄炎を起こした歯髄は、ほとんどの症例において、抜髄処置が施される。しかし、人工的に歯髄を再生させることが可能であるなら、歯の生活性が回復され、歯根破折などの抜歯の原因となる疾患を減らすことが可能となり、歯の寿命も延長すると考えられる。1980年代の終わり、化学者 Robert Langer らによって、足場に細胞を移植して組織を生じさせようという治療法が考案され（Scientific American 1995；273：130-133）、再生医学の礎となった。歯髄の再生においても、この組織再生の一般原理を応用できると考えられており、その原理に着目した研究が盛んに行われている。

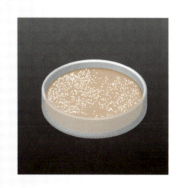

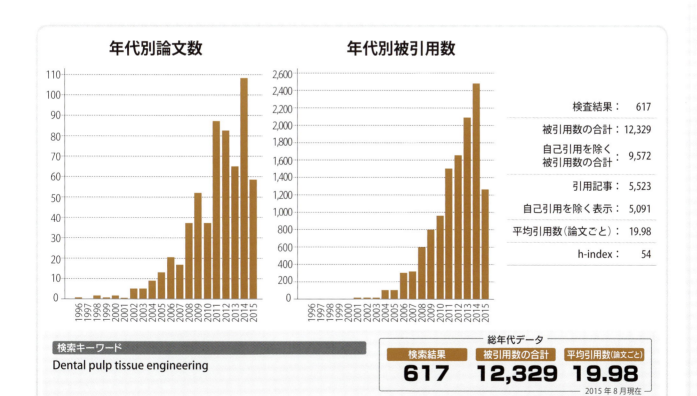

検査結果：　617
被引用数の合計：　12,329
自己引用を除く被引用数の合計：　9,572
引用記事：　5,523
自己引用を除く表示：　5,091
平均引用数（論文ごと）：　19.98
h-index：　54

検索キーワード
Dental pulp tissue engineering

総年代データ
検索結果 617　被引用数の合計 12,329　平均引用数（論文ごと） 19.98
2015 年 8 月現在

トムソン・ロイターが選んだベスト12論文

	タイトル・和訳	2011年	2012年	2013年	2014年	合計引用数
引用数 1位	Miura M, Gronthos S, Zhao M, Lu B, Fisher LW, Robey PG, Shi S. SHED: stem cells from human exfoliated deciduous teeth. Proc Natl Acad Sci USA 2003; 100(10): 5807-5812. SHED: ヒト脱落乳歯歯髄幹細胞 チャプター20に和訳あり	93	119	112	137	888
引用数 2位	Huang GT, Gronthos S, Shi S. Mesenchymal stem cells derived from dental tissues vs. those from other sources: Their biology and role in regenerative medicine. J Dent Res 2009; 88(9): 792-806. 歯系組織由来の間葉系幹細胞対その他組織の間葉系幹細胞：再生医療における間葉系幹細胞の生物学と役割 本項に和訳あり	62	81	91	94	399
引用数 3位	Young CS, Terada S, Vacanti JP, Honda M, Bartlett JD, Yelick PC. Tissue engineering of complex tooth structures on biodegradable polymer scaffolds. J Dent Res 2002; 81(10): 695-700. 生体吸収性ポリマーからなるスキャホールド（足場）を用いた歯の構造の組織工学 本項に和訳あり	26	23	13	17	239
引用数 4位	Shi S, Bartold PM, Miura M, Seo BM, Robey PG, Gronthos S. The efficacy of mesenchymal stem cells to regenerate and repair dental structures. Orthod Craniofac Res 2005; 8(3): 191-199. 歯の構造の再生と修復に対する間葉系幹細胞の有効性 本項に和訳あり	30	25	31	20	217
引用数 5位	Nakashima M, Reddi AH. The application of bone morphogenetic proteins to dental tissue engineering. Nat Biotechnol 2003; 21(9): 1025-1032. 歯の再生医療への骨形成タンパク質の応用	17	18	16	23	193
引用数 6位	Goldberg M, Smith AJ. Cells and extracellular matrices of dentin and pulp: A biological basis for repair and tissue engineering. Crit Rev Oral Biol Med 2004; 15(1): 13-27. 象牙質と歯髄の細胞および細胞外基質：修復と再生医学の生物学的根幹 本項に和訳あり	22	23	26	17	191
引用数 7位	Duailibi MT, Duailibi SE, Young CS, Bartlett JD, Vacanti JP, Yelick PC. Bioengineered teeth from cultured rat tooth bud cells. J Dent Res 2004; 83(7): 523-528. 培養ラット歯胚細胞からバイオエンジニアリングにより作製された歯 本項に和訳あり	21	15	18	9	181

19 Dental pulp tissue engineering

トムソン・ロイターが選んだベスト12論文

	タイトル・和訳	2011年	2012年	2013年	2014年	合計引用数
引用数 8位	Cordeiro MM, Dong Z, Kaneko T, Zhang Z, Miyazawa M, Shi S, Smith AJ, Nör JE. Dental pulp tissue engineering with stem cells from exfoliated deciduous teeth. J Endod 2008；34(8)：962-962. 脱落乳歯歯髄幹細胞を用いた歯髄組織工学	29	27	31	38	166
引用数 9位	Huang GT, Sonoyama W, Liu Y, Liu H, Wang S, Shi S. The hidden treasure in apical papilla：The potential role in pulp/dentin regeneration and bioroot engineering. J Endod 2008；34(6)：645-651. 歯乳頭に隠された宝：歯髄/象牙質の再生と再生歯根組織工学における潜在的役割	27	26	39	31	165
引用数 10位	Jo YY, Lee HJ, Kook SY, Choung HW, Park JY, Chung JH, Choung YH, Kim ES, Yang HC, Choung PH. Isolation and characterization of postnatal stem cells from human dental tissues. Tissue Eng 2007；13(4)：767-773. ヒト歯牙組織由来の成体幹細胞の単離と特性評価	31	30	22	14	146
引用数 11位	Gay IC, Chen S, MacDougall M. Isolation and characterization of multipotent human periodontal ligament stem cells. Orthod Craniofac Res 2007；10(3)：149-160. 多能性ヒト歯根膜幹細胞の単離と特性評価	19	28	23	23	143
引用数 12位	Nakashima M, Akamine A. The application of tissue engineering to regeneration of pulp and dentin in endodontics. J Endod 2005；31(10)：711-718. 歯内療法における歯髄および象牙質を再生するための組織工学の応用 **チャプター1に和訳あり**	17	11	16	15	122

Mesenchymal stem cells derived from dental tissues vs. those from other sources : Their biology and role in regenerative medicine.

歯系組織由来の間葉系幹細胞対その他組織の間葉系幹細胞：再生医療における間葉系幹細胞の生物学と役割

Huang GT, Gronthos S, Shi S.

　現在までに、歯髄幹細胞、脱落乳歯歯髄幹細胞、歯根膜幹細胞、歯乳頭幹細胞、および歯小嚢前駆細胞という5種の異なるヒト歯系幹細胞・前駆細胞が単離・同定されている。これらの成体幹細胞群は、自己複製能および多分化能を含んでおり、間葉系幹細胞に似た性質を有している。骨髄由来間葉系幹細胞は硬組織形成細胞、軟骨形成細胞、脂肪生成細胞、筋原細胞、そして神経細胞といったさまざまな系統の細胞になることができる。歯系組織由来幹細胞は、歯原性細胞へ分化するための高い能力を有する特殊な組織から単離される。しかし、歯系組織由来幹細胞は骨髄由来間葉系幹細胞と同じように他の細胞系統を生じる能力を有するが、骨髄由来間葉系幹細胞とは能力の点で異なっている。本論文では、歯系組織由来幹細胞様細胞の単離と機能的特徴を、骨髄由来間葉系幹細胞をはじめとするその他の間葉系幹細胞と比較して論評する。本論文では、幹細胞ニッチェ、ホーミング、そして免疫調整といった幹細胞生物学に関する重要な論点に関しても考察した。

（J Dent Res 2009 ; 88（9）: 792-806.）

To date, 5 different human dental stem/progenitor cells have been isolated and characterized: dental pulp stem cells (DPSCs), stem cells from exfoliated deciduous teeth (SHED), periodontal ligament stem cells (PDLSCs), stem cells from apical papilla (SCAP), and dental follicle progenitor cells (DFPCs). These postnatal populations have mesenchymal-stem-cell-like (MSC) qualities, including the capacity for self-renewal and multilineage differentiation potential. MSCs derived from bone marrow (BMMSCs) are capable of giving rise to various lineages of cells, such as osteogenic, chondrogenic, adipogenic, myogenic, and neurogenic cells. The dental-tissue-derived stem cells are isolated from specialized tissue with potent capacities to differentiate into odontogenic cells. However, they also have the ability to give rise to other cell lineages similar to, but different in potency from, that of BMMSCs. This article will review the isolation and characterization of the properties of different dental MSC-like populations in comparison with those of other MSCs, such as BMMSCs. Important issues in stem cell biology, such as stem cell niche, homing, and immunoregulation, will also be discussed.

Dental pulp tissue engineering

Tissue engineering of complex tooth structures on biodegradable polymer scaffolds.

生体吸収性ポリマーからなるスキャホールド（足場）を用いた歯の構造の組織工学

Young CS, Terada S, Vacanti JP, Honda M, Bartlett JD, Yelick PC.

　歯周病、う蝕、外傷、もしくは種々の遺伝性疾患による歯の喪失は、生活のある時点から、ほとんどの人に悪影響を及ぼし続けることになる。喪失歯に代わる生物学的な歯による補填は、現行の臨床治療にきわめて重要な代替治療案を提供するだろう。この目標を追求するため、われわれはブタの第三大臼歯の歯胚から細胞を単離し、生体吸収性ポリマーに播種した。これを宿主ラット内に20週から30週移植し、増殖させると、象牙質、象牙芽細胞、明確な髄室、ヘルトヴィッヒの上皮鞘と思われるもの、セメント芽細胞と思われるもの、そして完全形成されたエナメル質を含む形態学的に正常なエナメル器官を含む歯の構造物と認識可能な構造物を形成していた。われわれの結果は、単離した歯の組織から象牙質とエナメル質の両方を含む歯冠構造物再生の成功の第一段階であることを示し、そしてブタの第三大臼歯組織における上皮歯系幹細胞および間葉系歯系幹細胞の存在を示唆するものである。

（J Dent Res 2002；81(10)：695-700.）

Tooth loss due to periodontal disease, dental caries, trauma, or a variety of genetic disorders continues to affect most adults adversely at some time in their lives. A biological tooth substitute that could replace lost teeth would provide a vital alternative to currently available clinical treatments. To pursue this goal, we dissociated porcine third molar tooth buds into single-cell suspensions and seeded them onto biodegradable polymers. After growing in rat hosts for 20 to 30 weeks, recognizable tooth structures formed that contained dentin, odontoblasts, a well-defined pulp chamber, putative Hertwig's root sheath epithelia, putative cementoblasts, and a morphologically correct enamel organ containing fully formed enamel. Our results demonstrate the first successful generation of tooth crowns from dissociated tooth tissues that contain both dentin and enamel, and suggest the presence of epithelial and mesenchymal dental stem cells in porcine third molar tissues.

The efficacy of mesenchymal stem cells to regenerate and repair dental structures.

歯の構造の再生と修復に対する間葉系幹細胞の有効性

Shi S, Bartold PM, Miura M, Seo BM, Robey PG, Gronthos S.

目的：ヒト歯系組織由来間葉系幹細胞の同定、特性評価、および応用の可能性を検索する。

方法：ヒト正常埋伏第三大臼歯から歯髄および歯根膜を採取した。単細胞浮遊液を生成するため、採取された組織はコラゲナーゼ/ディスパーゼを用いて分解された。細胞は、20%ウシ胎児血清、2 mM L-グルタミン、100μM L-アスコルビン酸-2-リン酸添加α-MEM培養液で培養された。新鮮分離後、ex vivo において増殖させた細胞群の表現型（phenotype）を特性評価するために、Magnetic activated cell sorting 法および fluorescence activated cell sorting 法が用いられた。ハイドロキシアパタイト/リン酸三カルシウム（HA/TCP）複合体の小片とともに免疫不全マウスに8週間移植した後に、培養細胞の発生能力が評価された。

結果：培養条件下において採取された細胞にコロニー性細胞集塊形成能が認められたことから、ヒト永久歯歯髄（歯髄幹細胞）、ヒト乳歯（脱落乳歯歯髄幹細胞）、歯根膜（歯根膜幹細胞）において、間葉系幹細胞が同定された。ex vivo 下において増殖させた歯髄幹細胞、脱落乳歯歯髄幹細胞、歯根膜幹細胞群は、間葉系幹細胞、象牙質、骨、平滑筋、神経組織、内皮に関連したさまざまなマーカーを発現した。歯根膜幹細胞が、腱特異的マーカーである Scleraxis を発現することもわかった。歯髄幹細胞あるいは脱落乳歯歯髄幹細胞を混合した HA/TCP を含む異種間移植は、石灰化象牙質基質に沿って明確な象牙芽細胞層を有する宿主由来の象牙質/歯髄様組織を生じた。上述の実験に並行して行われた実験において、免疫不全マウスに HA/TCP 複合体を移植すると、歯根膜幹細胞は、歯根膜様結合組織に関連するセメント質様構造物を生じた。

結論：総括すると、これらのデータは、in vivo においてヒトの歯系生組織を再生するための歯系構造物や幹細胞能に関連した明確な間葉系幹細胞群の存在を明らかにしている。

（Orthod Craniofac Res 2005；8（3）：191-199.）

OBJECTIVES: Identification, characterization, and potential application of mesenchymal stem cells (MSC) derived from human dental tissues.
METHODS: Dental pulp and periodontal ligament were obtained from normal human impacted third molars. The tissues were digested in collagenase/dispase to generate single cell suspensions. Cells were cultured in alpha-MEM supplemented with 20% fetal bovine serum, 2 mM l-glutamine, 100 microM l-ascorbate-2-phosphate. Magnetic and fluorescence activated cell sorting were employed to characterize the phenotype of freshly isolated and ex vivo expanded cell populations. The developmental potential of cultured cells was assessed following co-transplantation with hydroxyapetite/tricalcium phosphate (HA/TCP) particles into immunocompromised mice for 8 weeks.
RESULTS: MSC were identified in adult human dental pulp (dental pulp stem cells, DPSC), human primary teeth (stem cells from human exfoliated deciduous teeth, SHED), and periodontal ligament (periodontal ligament stem cells, PDLSC) by their capacity to generate clongenic cell clusters in culture. Ex vivo expanded DPSC, SHED, and PDLSC populations expressed a heterogeneous assortment of makers associated with MSC, dentin, bone, smooth muscle, neural tissue, and endothelium. PDLSC were also found to express the tendon specific marker, Scleraxis. Xenogeneic transplants containing HA/TCP with either DPSC or SHED generated donor-derived dentin-pulp-like tissues with distinct odontoblast layers lining the mineralized dentin-matrix. In parallel studies, PDLSC generated cementum-like structures associated with PDL-like connective tissue when transplanted with HA/TCP into immunocompromised mice.
CONCLUSION: Collectively, these data revealed the presence of distinct MSC populations associated with dental structures with the potential of stem cells to regenerate living human dental tissues in vivo.

Dental pulp tissue engineering

Cells and extracellular matrices of dentin and pulp : A biological basis for repair and tissue engineering.

象牙質と歯髄の細胞および細胞外基質： 修復と再生医学の生物学的根幹

Goldberg M, Smith AJ.

象牙芽細胞は象牙質に観察され、象牙質の石灰化に関与する細胞外基質要素の大部分を産生する。なぜ歯髄は正常時に非石灰化組織なのかは、歯髄細胞外基質における大きな違いで説明できる。*in vitro* や *in vivo* において、いくつかの象牙質細胞外基質分子は結晶核形成に作用し、結晶成長に寄与する。一方、その他の象牙質細胞外基質分子は石灰化抑制物質である。中等度う蝕の治療後、象牙芽細胞と Höhl's 層（象牙芽細胞層の下層）の細胞は反応象牙質形成に関与する。歯髄に近接した深い象牙質病変の治癒は、歯髄細胞による修復象牙質形成を生じる。水酸化カルシウムのような材料を用いた直接覆髄に対する反応は、幹細胞や脱分化・形質転換した成熟細胞のような未分化細胞の動員・増殖が生じた結果、デンティンブリッジ形成となる。一度分化が生じると、その細胞は石灰化を起こす基質を合成する。生理活性分子の歯髄移植後の歯髄修復を促進する潜在的生理活性分子の能力を調査するために、実験動物モデルが用いられてきた。細胞外基質分子はデンティンブリッジ形成や冠部歯髄における広範囲の石灰化形成を誘導した。それらは、また、根管歯髄の完全閉塞の原因ともなる。結論として、象牙質細胞外基質中のいくつかの分子は、歯髄修復や再生医学に対しての生理活性材として、歯科治療における可能性を秘めているかもしれない。

（Crit Rev Oral Biol Med 2004；15(1)：13-27.）

Odontoblasts produce most of the extracellular matrix (ECM) components found in dentin and implicated in dentin mineralization. Major differences in the pulp ECM explain why pulp is normally a non-mineralized tissue. *In vitro* or *in vivo*, some dentin ECM molecules act as crystal nucleators and contribute to crystal growth, whereas others are mineralization inhibitors. After treatment of caries lesions of moderate progression, odontoblasts and cells from the sub-odontoblastic Höhl's layer are implicated in the formation of reactionary dentin. Healing of deeper lesions in contact with the pulp results in the formation of reparative dentin by pulp cells. The response to direct pulp-capping with materials such as calcium hydroxide is the formation of a dentinal bridge, resulting from the recruitment and proliferation of undifferentiated cells, which may be either stem cells or dedifferentiated and transdifferentiated mature cells. Once differentiated, the cells synthesize a matrix that undergoes mineralization. Animal models have been used to test the capacity of potentially bioactive molecules to promote pulp repair following their implantation into the pulp. ECM molecules induce either the formation of dentinal bridges or large areas of mineralization in the coronal pulp. They may also stimulate the total closure of the pulp in the root canal. In conclusion, some molecules found in dentin extracellular matrix may have potential in dental therapy as bioactive agents for pulp repair or tissue engineering.

Bioengineered teeth from cultured rat tooth bud cells.

培養ラット歯胚細胞から
バイオエンジニアリングにより作製された歯

Duailibi MT, Duailibi SE, Young CS, Bartlett JD, Vacanti JP, Yelick PC.

　ブタ歯胚組織から複合体的歯牙構造をつくるという最近のバイオエンジニアリングは、哺乳類における歯の組織再生への可能性を示唆するものである。われわれは、生後3日から7日の歯と組織の再生法を適用したラットから採取されたラット歯胚培養細胞の有用性を比較することから、歯の生物学的再生法の向上をはかった。細胞を播種した生体吸収性スキャホールド（足場）は、12週間宿主成熟ラットの腹部大網中で増殖後、摘出された。移植12週経過後の組織解析は、生後4日ラットから分離後、PGA あるいは PLGA スキャホールド（足場）に1時間播種した歯胚細胞はもっとも確実に再生歯系組織を形成することを示していた。われわれは、歯の組織再生法はブタ組織およびラット組織の再生に用いることが可能であると結論づけた。さらに、生物工学を用いて培養歯胚細胞から歯系構造を作るわれわれの技術は、歯の上皮細胞と間葉系幹細胞を少なくとも6日間 *in vitro* で維持可能であることを、示唆するものである。

（J Dent Res 2004；83（7）：523-528.）

The recent bioengineering of complex tooth structures from pig tooth bud tissues suggests the potential for the regeneration of mammalian dental tissues. We have improved tooth bioengineering methods by comparing the utility of cultured rat tooth bud cells obtained from three- to seven-day post-natal (dpn) rats for tooth-tissue-engineering applications. Cell-seeded biodegradable scaffolds were grown in the omenta of adult rat hosts for 12 wks, then harvested. Analyses of 12-week implant tissues demonstrated that dissociated 4-dpn rat tooth bud cells seeded for 1 hr onto PGA or PLGA scaffolds generated bioengineered tooth tissues most reliably. We conclude that tooth-tissue-engineering methods can be used to generate both pig and rat tooth tissues. Furthermore, our ability to bioengineer tooth structures from cultured tooth bud cells suggests that dental epithelial and mesenchymal stem cells can be maintained *in vitro* for at least 6 days.

エンドのための重要20キーワード

20 Dental pulp cells
歯髄細胞

歯髄は歯乳頭に由来した線維性結合組織であり、種々の細胞、血管、神経で満たされている。象牙芽細胞、線維芽細胞、あるいは歯髄の防御機構としての役割を担う免疫担当細胞などの他に、間葉系幹細胞が歯髄には存在することがわかっている。このような歯髄由来幹細胞に対する研究が現在多く行われており、歯髄再生療法の実現が期待されている。

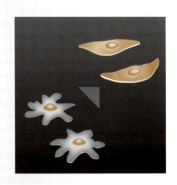

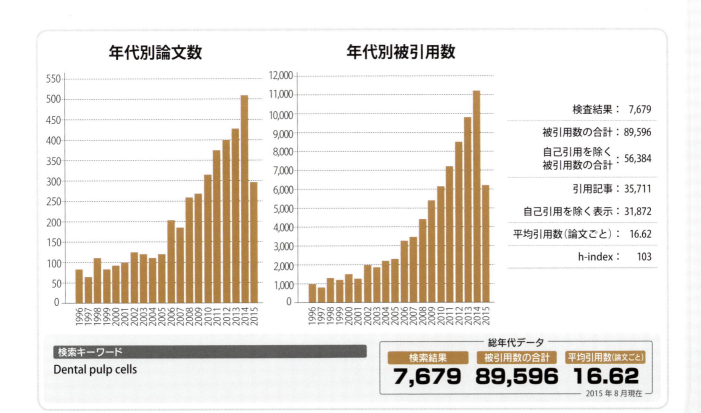

検索キーワード: Dental pulp cells

検査結果	7,679
被引用数の合計	89,596
自己引用を除く被引用数の合計	56,384
引用記事	35,711
自己引用を除く表示	31,872
平均引用数(論文ごと)	16.62
h-index	103

総年代データ
- 検索結果: 7,679
- 被引用数の合計: 89,596
- 平均引用数(論文ごと): 16.62

2015年8月現在

エンドのための重要20キーワード（関連性の高い論文和訳）

トムソン・ロイターが選んだベスト12論文

	タイトル・和訳	2011年	2012年	2013年	2014年	合計引用数
引用数1位	Gronthos S, Mankani M, Brahim J, Robey PG, Shi S. Postnatal human dental pulp stem cells (DPSCs) *in vitro* and *in vivo*. Proc Natl Acad Sci USA 2000；97(25)：13625-13630. *in vitro* および *in vivo* におけるヒト成体歯髄幹細胞 本項に和訳あり	174	169	192	209	1,390
引用数2位	Seo BM, Miura M, Gronthos S, Bartold PM, Batouli S, Brahim J, Young M, Robey PG, Wang CY, Shi S. Investigation of multipotent postnatal stem cells from human periodontal ligament. Lancet 2004；364(9429)：149-155. ヒト歯根膜由来の多能性成体幹細胞に関する研究	107	140	172	170	1,006
引用数3位	Miura M, Gronthos S, Zhao M, Lu B, Fisher LW, Robey PG, Shi S. SHED：stem cells from human exfoliated deciduous teeth. Proc Natl Acad Sci USA 2003；100(10)：5807-5812. SHED：ヒト脱落乳歯歯髄幹細胞 本項に和訳あり	93	119	112	137	888
引用数4位	Gronthos S, Brahim J, Li W, Fisher LW, Cherman N, Boyde A, DenBesten P, Robey PG, Shi S. Stem cell properties of human dental pulp stem cells. J Dent Res 2002；81(8)：531-535. ヒト歯髄幹細胞の幹細胞特性 本項に和訳あり	85	86	92	93	734
引用数5位	Shi S, Gronthos S. Perivascular niche of postnatal mesenchymal stem cells in human bone marrow and dental pulp. J Bone Miner Res 2003；18(4)：696-704. ヒト骨髄および歯髄における成体間葉系幹細胞の血管周囲ニッチェ	77	84	87	63	654
引用数6位	Huang GT, Gronthos S, Shi S. Mesenchymal stem cells derived from dental tissues vs. those from other sources：Their biology and role in regenerative medicine. J Dent Res 2009；88(9)：792-806. 歯性組織由来の間葉系幹細胞対その他の組織由来の間葉系幹細胞：再生医療における間葉系幹細胞の生物学と役割 チャプター19に和訳あり	62	81	91	94	399
引用数7位	Nair PN, Sjögren U, Krey G, Kahnberg KE, Sundqvist G. Intraradicular bacteria and fungi in root-filled, asymptomatic human teeth with therapy-resistant periapical lesions：a long-term light and electron microscopic follow-up study. J Endod 1990；16(12)：580-588. 治療耐性を有した根尖病巣の認められるヒト無症状根管充填歯における根管内細菌および真菌：長期にわたる光学および電子顕微鏡による追跡研究	12	12	10	15	277

20 Dental pulp cells

トムソン・ロイターが選んだベスト12論文

	タイトル・和訳	2011年	2012年	2013年	2014年	合計引用数
引用数 8位	Sonoyama W, Liu Y, Yamaza T, Tuan RS, Wang S, Shi S, Huang GT. Characterization of the apical papilla and its residing stem cells from human immature permanent teeth：a pilot study. J Endod 2008；34(2)：166-171. ヒト幼若永久歯由来の歯乳頭と歯乳頭幹細胞の特性評価：予備実験 **チャプター18に和訳あり**	46	46	58	60	277
引用数 9位	Schröder U. Effects of calcium hydroxide-containing pulp-capping agents on pulp cell migration, proliferation, and differentiation. J Dent Res 1985；64：541-548. 歯髄細胞の遊走、増殖、および分化に対する水酸化カルシウム含有覆髄材の効果	8	16	13	15	243
引用数 10位	Tziafas D, Smith AJ, Lesot H. Designing new treatment strategies in vital pulp therapy. J Dent 2000；28(2)：77-92. 生活歯髄療法における新しい治療の設計戦略	17	15	11	10	203
引用数 11位	Batouli S, Miura M, Brahim J, Tsutsui TW, Fisher LW, Gronthos S, Robey PG, Shi S. Comparison of stem-cell-mediated osteogenesis and dentinogenesis. J Dent Res 2003；82(12)：976-981. 幹細胞を介した骨再生と象牙質再生の比較 **本項に和訳あり**	24	20	18	16	183
引用数 12位	Yamamura T. Differentiation of pulpal cells and inductive influences of various matrices with reference to pulpal wound healing. J Dent Res 1985；64：530-540. 歯髄の創傷治癒と関連した歯髄細胞の分化と種々の基質の誘導的影響 **本項に和訳あり**	7	8	1	2	154

Postnatal human dental pulp stem cells (DPSCs) *in vitro* and *in vivo*.

in vitro および *in vivo* におけるヒト成体歯髄幹細胞

Gronthos S, Mankani M, Brahim J, Robey PG, Shi S.

　生体組織における象牙質修復はいまだ同定されていないが、前駆細胞群により維持されていると思われる特異的細胞、および象牙芽細胞の活動を通じて起こる。本研究では、われわれはヒト成体歯髄組織由来のクローン原性と迅速な増殖能を有する細胞群を単離した。その後、これら歯髄幹細胞は骨芽細胞の前駆細胞として知られるヒト骨髄間質細胞と比較された。*in vitro* において両者の細胞は同様な免疫表現型を共有しているものの、細胞機能の実験は、以下の結果を示していた。具体的には、歯髄幹細胞は脂肪細胞にはならずに、散発的であるが高密度な石灰化結節を生じ、一方、骨髄間質細胞は、脂質を含有した脂肪細胞のクラスター形成を認める付着細胞層全域でつねに石灰化を生じていた。歯髄幹細胞を免疫不全マウスに移植すると、歯髄幹細胞は、歯髄様間質組織の表層にヒト象牙芽細胞様細胞が並ぶ象牙質様構造を形成した。対照的に、骨髄間質細胞は、活性化した新生血球や脂肪細胞をともなった線維性脈管組織に骨細胞を含み、その表層に骨芽細胞が並ぶ層板骨を形成した。本研究により象牙質/歯髄複合体を形成するための能力を有するヒト成体歯髄幹細胞が単離された。

（Proc Natl Acad Sci USA 2000；97(25)：13625-13630.）

Dentinal repair in the postnatal organism occurs through the activity of specialized cells, odontoblasts, that are thought to be maintained by an as yet undefined precursor population associated with pulp tissue. In this study, we isolated a clonogenic, rapidly proliferative population of cells from adult human dental pulp. These DPSCs were then compared with human bone marrow stromal cells (BMSCs), known precursors of osteoblasts. Although they share a similar immunophenotype *in vitro*, functional studies showed that DPSCs produced only sporadic, but densely calcified nodules, and did not form adipocytes, whereas BMSCs routinely calcified throughout the adherent cell layer with clusters of lipid-laden adipocytes. When DPSCs were transplanted into immunocompromised mice, they generated a dentin-like structure lined with human odontoblast-like cells that surrounded a pulp-like interstitial tissue. In contrast, BMSCs formed lamellar bone containing osteocytes and surface-lining osteoblasts, surrounding a fibrous vascular tissue with active hematopoiesis and adipocytes. This study isolates postnatal human DPSCs that have the ability to form a dentin/pulp-like complex.

20 Dental pulp cells

SHED：stem cells from human exfoliated deciduous teeth.

SHED：ヒト脱落乳歯歯髄幹細胞

Miura M, Gronthos S, Zhao M, Lu B, Fisher LW, Robey PG, Shi S.

　入手の容易なリソース由来の良質なヒト成体幹細胞を単離することが幹細胞研究の重要目標である。本研究においてわれわれは、脱落ヒト乳歯が多能性幹細胞（ヒト脱落乳歯幹細胞）を含むことを見出した。ヒト脱落乳歯幹細胞は、神経細胞、脂肪細胞、および象牙芽細胞を含むさまざまな細胞種へ分化可能な高増殖能のクローン化可能細胞群として同定された。in vivo においてヒト脱落乳歯幹細胞を移植すると、ヒト脱落乳歯幹細胞は骨形成や象牙質を生じ、そして神経マーカーを発現しながらマウスの脳でも生き抜くことがわかった。ここにわれわれは、自然脱落したヒト器官がいままで同定された幹細胞とは完全に異なる幹細胞群を含むことを結論づけた。ヒト脱落乳歯幹細胞は入手の容易な組織リソース由来であるだけでなく、臨床応用への潜在能力を有した十分な細胞数量を供給可能である。すなわち、脱落歯は、自己幹細胞移植や組織工学という幹細胞療法における予想せぬユニークなリソースであるかもしれない。

（Proc Natl Acad Sci USA 2003；100（10）：5807-5812.）

To isolate high-quality human postnatal stem cells from accessible resources is an important goal for stem-cell research. In this study we found that exfoliated human deciduous tooth contains multipotent stem cells [stem cells from human exfoliated deciduous teeth (SHED)]. SHED were identified to be a population of highly proliferative, clonogenic cells capable of differentiating into a variety of cell types including neural cells, adipocytes, and odontoblasts. After *in vivo* transplantation, SHED were found to be able to induce bone formation, generate dentin, and survive in mouse brain along with expression of neural markers. Here we show that a naturally exfoliated human organ contains a population of stem cells that are completely different from previously identified stem cells. SHED are not only derived from a very accessible tissue resource but are also capable of providing enough cells for potential clinical application. Thus, exfoliated teeth may be an unexpected unique resource for stem-cell therapies including autologous stem-cell transplantation and tissue engineering.

Stem cell properties of human dental pulp stem cells.

ヒト歯髄幹細胞の幹細胞特性

Gronthos S, Brahim J, Li W, Fisher LW, Cherman N, Boyde A, DenBesten P, Robey PG, Shi S.

　本研究において、われわれはヒト歯髄幹細胞の自己複製能、多分化能、およびコロニー形成率を明らかにした。*in vivo* において、歯髄幹細胞は異所性象牙質および歯髄関連組織の形成が可能であった。歯髄幹細胞に自己複製能があることを証明することを目的として、間質様細胞を歯髄幹細胞の初代移植組織から培養条件下で再樹立し、象牙質-歯髄様組織再生のため、免疫不全マウスに再び移植した。歯髄幹細胞は、脂肪細胞と神経様細胞に分化できることもわかった。それぞれが歯原性組織になる可能性を有する単集落由来の歯髄幹細胞株12株が同定された。*in vivo* において、単集落由来の歯髄幹細胞株の2/3が大量の異所性象牙質を生じたが、一方、残りの1/3の歯髄幹細胞株ではごく少量の象牙質しか生じなかった。これらの結果から、単集落由来歯髄幹細胞株は象牙質形成率がそれぞれ異なることが示された。これらの結果をまとめると、歯髄幹細胞は自己複製能と多分化能という幹細胞様の性質を有していることがわかった。

（J Dent Res 2002；81（8）：531-535.）

In this study, we characterized the self-renewal capability, multi-lineage differentiation capacity, and clonogenic efficiency of human dental pulp stem cells (DPSCs). DPSCs were capable of forming ectopic dentin and associated pulp tissue *in vivo*. Stromal-like cells were reestablished in culture from primary DPSC transplants and re-transplanted into immunocompromised mice to generate a dentin-pulp-like tissue, demonstrating their self-renewal capability. DPSCs were also found to be capable of differentiating into adipocytes and neural-like cells. The odontogenic potential of 12 individual single-colony-derived DPSC strains was determined. Two-thirds of the single-colony-derived DPSC strains generated abundant ectopic dentin *in vivo*, while only a limited amount of dentin was detected in the remaining one-third. These results indicate that single-colony-derived DPSC strains differ from each other with respect to their rate of odontogenesis. Taken together, these results demonstrate that DPSCs possess stem-cell-like qualities, including self-renewal capability and multi-lineage differentiation.

Dental pulp cells

Comparison of stem-cell-mediated osteogenesis and dentinogenesis.

幹細胞を介した骨再生と象牙質再生の比較

Batouli S, Miura M, Brahim J, Tsutsui TW, Fisher LW, Gronthos S, Robey PG, Shi S.

　幹細胞を介した骨再生と象牙質再生の相違はいまだよくわかっていない。本論文において、骨髄間質幹細胞と歯髄幹細胞との間の調節機構の相違を研究するため、*in vivo* 幹細胞移植実験系をわれわれは採用した。basic fibroblast growth factor と matrix metalloproteinase 9 の発現上昇が、骨髄間質幹細胞を移植した組織の造血髄形成に関連して観察されたが、歯髄幹細胞を移植した組織の結合組織では観察されなかった。dentin sialoprotein の発現は、歯髄幹細胞を移植組織内に形成された象牙質においてとくに認められた。さらに、歯髄幹細胞は *in vivo* においてヒト象牙質表面に修復象牙質様組織を形成できることがわかった。本研究は、骨髄間質幹細胞を介した骨形成と歯髄幹細胞を介した象牙質形成のそれぞれが、石灰化組織、そして非石灰化組織という別の組織という異なった仕組みにより制御されていることを示唆する直接的な根拠を与えるものであった。

（J Dent Res 2003；82(12)：976-981.）

The difference between stem-cell-mediated bone and dentin regeneration is not yet well-understood. Here we use an *in vivo* stem cell transplantation system to investigate differential regulation mechanisms of bone marrow stromal stem cells (BMSSCs) and dental pulp stem cells (DPSCs). Elevated expression of basic fibroblast growth factor (bFGF) and matrix metalloproteinase 9 (MMP-9, gelatinase B) was found to be associated with the formation of hematopoietic marrow in BMSSC transplants, but not in the connective tissue of DPSC transplants. The expression of dentin sialoprotein (DSP) specifically marked dentin synthesis in DPSC transplants. Moreover, DPSCs were found to be able to generate reparative dentin-like tissue on the surface of human dentin *in vivo*. This study provided direct evidence to suggest that osteogenesis and dentinogenesis mediated by BMSSCs and DPSCs, respectively, may be regulated by distinct mechanisms, leading to the different organization of the mineralized and non-mineralized tissues.

Differentiation of pulpal cells and inductive influences of various matrices with reference to pulpal wound healing.

歯髄の創傷治癒と関連した歯髄細胞の分化と種々の基質の誘導的影響

Yamamura T.

　近年の文献に基づいて、デンティンブリッジの形成に関与する新生象牙芽細胞の起源、ならびにさまざまな組織や基質に移植された間葉系細胞の動態を本総説で説明する。歯髄、骨膜、軟骨膜、処置象牙質、および骨基質の移植に関連した実験が、これら細胞の硬組織形成能を明らかにするために実施された。光学顕微鏡、電子顕微鏡、そしてオートラジオグラフィを用いた研究が、置き換わった象牙芽細胞の由来を明らかにするために実施された。歯髄細胞、内皮細胞、そして周皮細胞は、露髄後に未分化間葉系細胞になったと思われた。これらの間葉系細胞は、分化後に象牙質基質を産生する象牙芽細胞に分化した。歯髄と異なる部位に自家移植を行った歯髄組織は、骨基質（あるいは骨様象牙質）を産生したが、細管象牙質とは結合しなかった。無菌ラットを用いたデンティンブリッジの形成実験は、歯髄組織が固有の治癒能を有することを示していた。したがって、硬組織を生じるという歯髄組織の能力は、歯髄組織の置かれた環境によると結論づけられた。

（J Dent Res 1985 ; 64 : 530-540.）

Based on recent literature, the dynamics of mesenchymal cells in transplantation of various tissues and matrices, as well as the origin of new odontoblasts which participate in the formation of the dentin bridge, are described. Experiments involving implantation of pulp, periosteum, perichondrium, treated dentin, and bone matrices were performed to emphasize the capability of these cells to produce hard tissue. Light and electron microscopic and autoradiographic studies were carried out to clarify the origin of replacement odontoblasts. It appears that the pulp cells, endothelial cells, and pericytes become undifferentiated mesenchymal cells following pulp exposure. These mesenchymal cells differentiate into odontoblasts, which subsequently produce a dentin matrix. Pulp tissues autografted to non-pulpal sites, elaborated bone (or osteodentin) matrix, but they did not graft to tubular dentin. An experiment on dentin bridge formation, using germ-free rats, demonstrated that the pulp tissue has intrinsic healing potential. Therefore, it was concluded that the ability of pulp tissue to elaborate hard tissues depends on its environment.

講演や雑誌でよく見る、あの分類および文献

1. 根管形態の分類 — PAGE 160
2. イスムス形態の分類 — PAGE 162
3. 上顎第一大臼歯近心頬側根 — PAGE 164
4. 上顎第一大臼歯近心舌側根管の探知 — PAGE 165
5. 下顎大臼歯近心中央根管について — PAGE 166
6. 受動的超音波洗浄法 — PAGE 167
7. 臨床所見に基づく根尖性歯周組織疾患の分類 — PAGE 168
8. 根尖部エックス線透過像と歯内療法の成功率 — PAGE 169
9. 外傷歯破折の分類 — PAGE 170
10. 亀裂歯の分類 — PAGE 171
11. 根尖外科手術1年後のエックス線写真所見 — PAGE 172
12. 歯内療法における微生物 — PAGE 173
13. 細菌関連物質 — PAGE 174
14. 幹細胞のタンパクおよび遺伝子のプロフィール — PAGE 175

講演や雑誌でよく見る、あの分類および文献

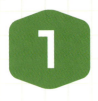 **根管形態の分類**

出典 Weine FS, Healey HJ, Gerstein H, Evanson L. Canal configuration in the mesiobuccal root of the maxillary first molar and its endodontic significance. Oral Surg Oral Med Oral Pathol 1969 ; 28 : 419–425.
Ballullaya SV, Vemuri S, Kumar PR. Variable permanent mandibular first molar : Review of literature. J Conserv Dent 2013 ; 16（2）: 99-110.
Vertucci FJ. Root canal anatomy of the human permanent teeth. Oral Surg Oral Med Oral Pathol 1984 ; 58 : 589–599.
Von Arx T. Frequency and type of canal isthmuses in first molars detected by endoscopic inspection during periradicular surgery. Int Endod J 2005 ; 38 : 160–168.

（1）Weine らによる根管形態の分類（Weine FS ら、Ballullaya SV らより改変引用）

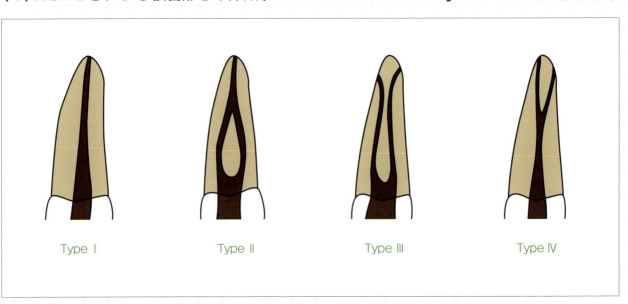

Type Ⅰ：1つの根管口－1つの根尖。
Type Ⅱ：2つの根管口－1つの根尖。
Type Ⅲ：2つの根管口－2つの根尖。
Type Ⅳ：1つの根管口－2つの根尖。

講演や雑誌でよく見る、あの分類および文献

（2）Vertucciらによる根管形態の分類（Vertucci FJ、Ballullaya SV らより改変引用）

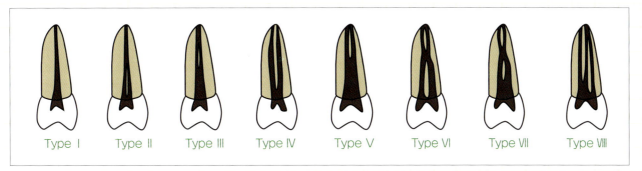

Type Ⅰ：1つの根管口－1つの根尖。
Type Ⅱ：2つの根管口－1つの根尖。
Type Ⅲ：1つの根管口－根管途中で2根管に分離－1つの根尖。
Type Ⅳ：2つの根管口－2つの根尖。
Type Ⅴ：1つの根管口－2つの根尖。
Type Ⅵ：2つの根管口－1つの根管に合流－2つの根尖。
Type Ⅶ：1つの根管口－根管途中で2根管に分離し、再度1根管に合流－2つの根尖。
Type Ⅷ：3つの根管口－3つの根尖。

（3）Von Arxによる根管形態の分類（Von Arx T、Ballullaya SV らより改変引用）

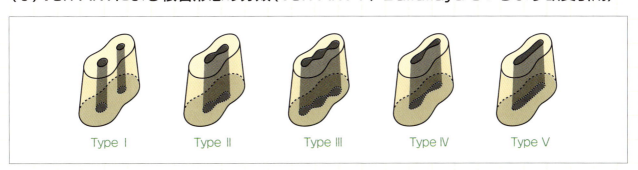

Type Ⅰ：2つの独立した根管。
Type Ⅱ：1つのイスムスで融合した2つの独立した根管。
Type Ⅲ：1つのイスムスで融合した3つの独立した根管。
Type Ⅳ：中心で融合した2つの細長い根管。
Type Ⅴ：幅広で細長い単根。

解説者コメント：根管は多様な解剖学的形態を有するが、WeineらやVertucciら、Von Arxは、根管形態を以上のように分類した。

講演や雑誌でよく見る、あの分類および文献

2 イスムス形態の分類

出典 Cohen S, Hargreaves KM・eds. Pathways of the pulp. 9 th ed. St Louis：Mosby-Elsevier, 2005.
Gu L, Wei X, Ling J, Huang X. A microcomputed tomographic study of canal isthmuses in the mesial root of mandibular first molars in a Chinese population. J Endod 2009；35(3)：353-356.

(1) 歯根水平断面におけるイスムス形態の分類
（Cohen S, Hargreaves KM・eds より改変引用）

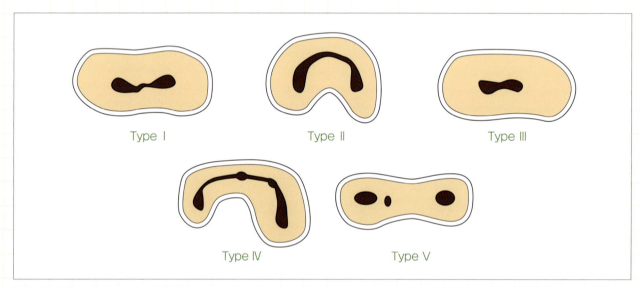

歯根水平断面におけるイスムス形態。

Type Ⅰ：不完全なイスムスであり、2つの根管にかすかなつながりがある。
Type Ⅱ：2つ根管をつなぐ明瞭なイスムス。
Type Ⅲ：2つの根管をつなぐ非常に短い、完全なイスムス。
Type Ⅳ：3つ以上の根管をつなぐ完全なイスムスや不完全なイスムス。
Type Ⅴ：2つもしくは3つの根管口を認めるが、根管間の交通は確認できない

解説者コメント：イスムスとは歯髄組織を含有し、根管同士が交通している狭窄部分のことである。イスムスへのアクセスは非常に困難であり、根管治療を行った後の予後不良の原因となる。

（2）マイクロ CT により解析を行った下顎第一大臼歯近心根のイスムス形態の分類
（Gu らより改変引用）

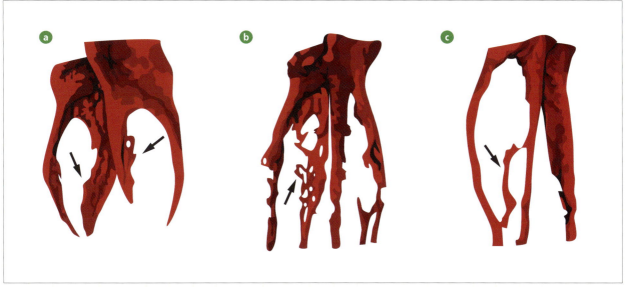

三次元解析によるイスムス形態の分類。ⓐ Fin-shaped isthmus、ⓑ Web-shaped isthmus、ⓒ Ribbon-shaped isthmus。

①1つの根管からイスムスへと伸びるフィン状の形態（Fin-shaped isthmus）。
②不規則に伸び，イスムス部分で根管が融合することにより、複雑かつ相互に連結した網状の形態（Web-shaped isthmus）。
③2つの主根管の間をつなぐ、明瞭な紐状の形態（Ribbon-shaped isthmus）。

解説者コメント：イスムスの形態に関する調査として、透明根管モデルや歯根の切断断面を評価したものが過去に報告されている。近年、マイクロ CT を用いて三次元的に根管形態を調査した研究が増加しており、本来の構造を保ったまま、任意の断面を検索可能となった。

講演や雑誌でよく見る、あの分類および文献

3 上顎第一大臼歯近心頰側根

出典 Weine FS, Hayami S, Hata G, Toda T. Canal configuration of the mesiobuccal root of the maxillary first molar of a Japanese sub-population. Int Endod J 1999；32（2）：79-87.

日本人における近心頰側根の根管形態

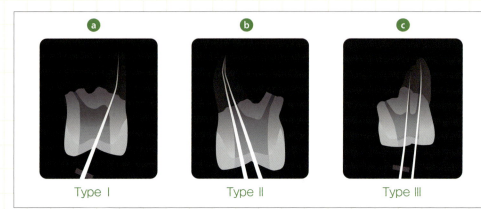
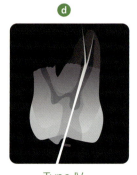

a　Type Ⅰ　　b　Type Ⅱ　　c　Type Ⅲ　　d　Type Ⅳ

上顎第一大臼歯の頰側遠心根。口蓋根を切断し、頰側根管にファイルを挿入した状態でのエックス線写真。

根管の分類	%
Type Ⅰ	42.0
Type Ⅱ	24.2
Type Ⅲ	30.4
Type Ⅳ	3.4
合計	100.0

日本人の上顎第一大臼歯頰側根293歯について、近心頰側根を根管形態に従い分類したときの各根管形態の発現率。

Type Ⅰ：1根管口－1根尖孔。
Type Ⅱ：2根管口－1根尖孔。
Type Ⅲ：2根管口－2根尖孔。
Type Ⅳ：1根管口－2根尖孔。
解説者コメント：上顎第一大臼歯近心頰側根は、日本人のおよそ60％で2根管性である。とくに、根尖側で分岐する場合は、根管探索に加え、根管形成や根管充填も非常に困難である。

4 上顎第一大臼歯近心舌側根管の探知

出典 Baldassari-Cruz LA, Lilly JP, Rivera EM. The influence of dental operating microscope in locating the mesiolingual canal orifice. Oral Surg Oral Med Oral Pathol Oral Radiol Endod 2002 ; 93（2）: 190-194.
Stropko JJ. Canal morphology of maxillary molars : clinical observations of canal configurations. J Endod 1999 ; 25（6）: 446-450.

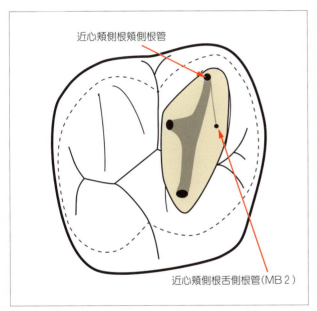

上顎第一大臼歯の根管口の模式図。

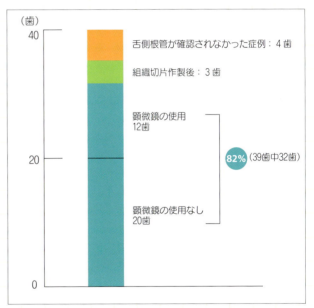

顕微鏡不使用、顕微鏡使用、そして組織切片作製により、確認された上顎第一大臼歯近心頬側根の舌側根管の発見歯数。顕微鏡を使用すると、MB2の発見率が上昇することがわかる。

解説者コメント：Baldassariら（2002）は、歯科用実体顕微鏡を使用することで上顎第一大臼歯近心頬側根の舌側根管（MB2）の発現率が上昇することを報告している。また、Stropko（1999）は、顕微鏡を使用するとMB2の発見率は上顎第一大臼歯で93％、第二大臼歯で60.4％であったと報告している。

講演や雑誌でよく見る、あの分類および文献

5 下顎大臼歯近心中央根管について

出典 Nosrat A, Deschenes RJ, Tordik PA, Hicks ML, Fouad AF. Middle mesial canals in mandibular molars：incidence and related factors. J Endod 2015；41(1)：28-32.
Pomeranz HH, Eidelman DL, Goldberg MG. Treatment considerations of the middle mesial canal of mandibular first and second molars. J Endod 1981；7(12)：565-568.

下顎大臼歯近心根の中央根管の形態分類（Nosratらより改変引用）

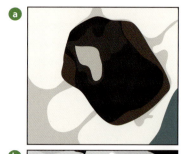
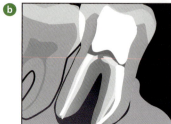
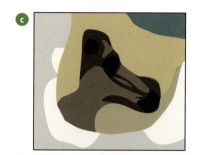
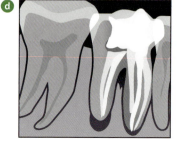
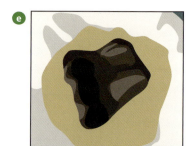
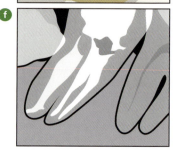

ⓐ、ⓑフィン状：近心舌側根管あるいは近心頰側根管と近心中央根管との間に交通がある。 ⓒ、ⓓ融合型：根管口では独立しているが、根尖付近で近心頰側根管あるいは近心舌側根管と近心中央根管とが合流する。 ⓔ、ⓕ独立型：根管口から根尖に至るまで、近心中央根管が独立している。

解説者コメント：Pomeranzら(1981)は、下顎大臼歯近心根の中央根管の根管形態の分類を、①フィン状(fin)、②融合型(confluent)、③独立型(independent)の3つのタイプに分類している。

6 受動的超音波洗浄法

出典 van der Sluis LW, Versluis M, Wu MK, Wesselink PR. Passive ultrasonic irrigation of the root canal：a review of the literature. Int Endod J 2007；40(6)：415-426.

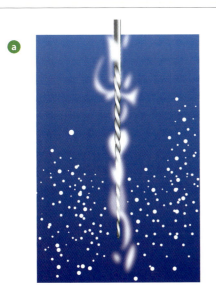 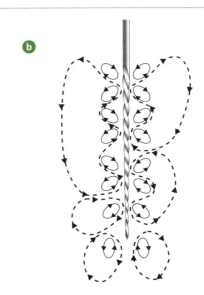

水のなかで受動的超音波洗浄法を行った際の超音波ファイル周囲の音響流（ⓐ）とその模式図（ⓑ）。

解説者コメント：歯内治療における超音波の使用は、1957年、Richman が超音波ファイルを用いて機械的に根管形成を行う可能性を示唆したことに始まる。この超音波ファイルを用いた根管形成法は、根尖部にパーフォレーションを起こしやすく、かつ根管形成の形状をコントロールすることが困難であった。その一方で，根管洗浄に超音波ファイルを用いることの臨床的意義は大きく、これまでに数多くの研究が報告されている。超音波を用いる根管洗浄法は、直接象牙質に超音波振動針を接して洗浄を行う方法（simultaneous ultrasonic instrumentation）と、超音波振動針を象牙質に直接触れずに洗浄を行う受動的超音波洗浄法（passive ultrasonic irrigation）に大別される。受動的超音波洗浄法の原理は，根管に挿入されたファイル周囲の洗浄液にキャビテーションが生じるためと考えられている。

講演や雑誌でよく見る、あの分類および文献

7 臨床所見に基づく根尖性歯周組織疾患の分類

出典 Hargreaves KM, Berman LH. Cohen's Pathways of the Pulp Expert Consult, 10th Edition. St Luis：Mosby, 2010.

臨床所見に基づく根尖性歯周組織疾患の分類

分類	臨床症状	根尖歯周組織の異常エックス線写真所見
正常根尖歯周組織	なし	なし
症状のある根尖性歯周炎	自発痛、打診痛	あり
症状のない根尖性歯周炎	なし	あり
急性根尖膿瘍	自発痛、打診痛、歯の動揺、腫脹など	あり
慢性根尖膿瘍	瘻孔形成、打診による違和感	あり

解説者コメント：2013年に米国歯内療法学会（以下、AAEと略）では、臨床症状とエックス線写真所見に基づき、上記の表のように根尖歯周組織疾患を5つに分類している。

8 根尖部エックス線透過像と歯内療法の成功率

出典 Sjogren U, Hagglund B, Sundqvist G, Wing K. Factors affecting the long-term results of endodontic treatment. J Endod 1990; 16(10): 498-504.

初発症例		再根管治療	
透過像なし	透過像あり	透過像なし	透過像あり
100%（102/102歯）	86%（176/204歯）	98%（169/173歯）	62%（58/94歯）

術前における根尖部エックス線透過像の有無と歯内療法の成功率の関係。根尖透過像のある症例では、透過像のない症例と比較して成功率が減少している。

解説者コメント：Sjogrenら（1990）は、歯内療法を施した8～10年後にその長期予後を評価し、治療の成否を評価するとともに、治療の成否に影響する因子について報告した（チャプター15に和訳あり）。

講演や雑誌でよく見る、あの分類および文献

 外傷歯破折の分類

出典 Clokie C, Metcalf I, Holland A. Dental trauma in anaesthesia. Can J Anaesth 1989；36(6)：675-680.
Cohen RC, Burns RC. Pathways to the pulp. St Louis：CV Mosby, 1980.

外傷歯破折の各分類におけるおおよその破折線（Clokie C らより改変引用）

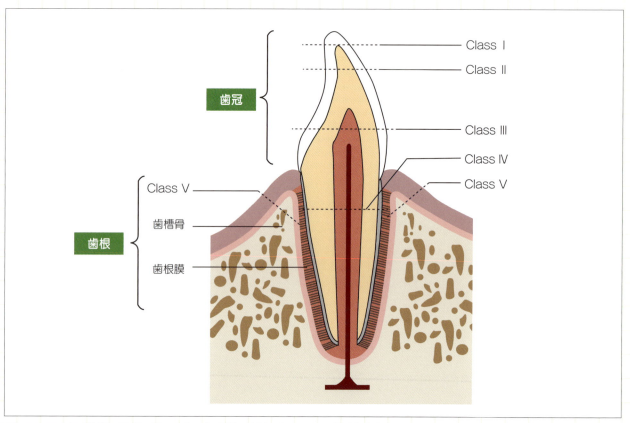

Class Ⅰ：エナメル質の破折、Class Ⅱ：象牙質の破折、Class Ⅲ：歯髄を含む破折、Class Ⅳ：歯根破折、Class Ⅴ：亜脱臼、Class Ⅵ：完全脱臼。Class Ⅴはたいてい歯根破折ではなく、歯槽骨折を生じる。Class Ⅵはたいてい脱臼のみで、歯根破折や骨折は認められない。

解説者コメント：外傷歯の破折（Cohen RC ら 1980）は、大きく図の 6 タイプに分類される。

10 亀裂歯の分類

出典 Kahler W. The cracked tooth conundrum：terminology, classification, diagnosis, and management. Am J Dent 2008；21（5）：275-282.

AAEによる破折歯の分類

分類	発生部位	方向	症状	歯髄の状態	予後
Craze lines	歯冠	多様	なし	生活	かなりよい
Fractured cusp	歯冠	近遠心または頬舌	咬合時と冷温に軽度の症状	たいてい生活	良
Cracked tooth	歯冠と歯根	近遠心 しばしば中心的	咬合時の急性症状 ときに冷温に対してするどい痛み	さまざま	疑わしい 破損の深さによる
Split tooth	歯冠と歯根	近遠心	咀嚼時の著しい痛み	根管充填歯の場合が多い	不良
Vertical root fracture	歯根	頬舌	漠然とした痛み 辺縁性歯周炎に類似した症状	ほとんどが根管充填歯	不良

解説者コメント：亀裂は主に歯冠や歯根の長軸方向に生じるが、破折の及ぶ方向、そして範囲はその後の治療の選択に重要である。そのため、明瞭化された破折歯の分類が診断に重要であることをAAEは報告している。

講演や雑誌でよく見る、あの分類および文献

11 根尖外科手術1年後のエックス線写真所見

出典 Molven O, Halse A, Grung B. Incomplete healing(scar tissue)after periapical surgery-radiographic findings 8 to 12 years after treatment. J Endod 1996；22(5)：264-268.

根尖外科手術1年後のエックス線写真による治癒評価の分類（Molvenらより改変引用）

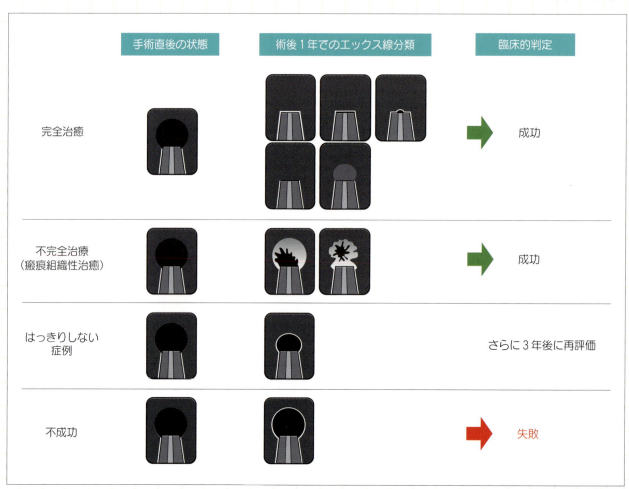

解説者コメント： Molvenら(1996)は、根尖部外科手術後のエックス線写真による治癒評価の分類を示した。治癒評価は術後1年で通常可能であることを報告している。

歯内療法における微生物

出典 Narayanan LL, Vaishnavi C. Endodontic microbiology. J Conserv Dent 2010;13(4):233-239.

歯内療法において観察される細菌

黒色色素産生性嫌気性グラム陰性桿菌	*Prevotella* *Prevotella intermedia、Prevotella nigrescens、Prevotella tannerae、Prevotella multissacharivorax、Prevotella baroniae and Prevotella denticola* *Porphyromonas* *Porphyromonas endodontalis、Porphyromonas gingivalis*
タネレラフォーサイシア (グラム陰性偏性嫌気性細菌)	
ジアリスタ属	*Dialister pneumosintes、Dialister invisus*
フソバクテリウム属	*Fusobacterium nucleatum、Fusobacterium periodonticum*
スピロヘータ	*Treponema denticola、Treponema sacranskii、Treponema parvum、Treponema maltophilum、Treponema lecithinolyticum*
グラム陽性嫌気性桿菌	*Pseudoramibacter alactolyticus、Filifactor alocis、Actinomyces spp、Propionibacterium propionicum、Olsenella spp、Slackia exigua、Mogibacterium timidum and Eubacterium spp*
グラム陰性球菌	*Parvimonas micra、Streptococcus spp(Streptococcus anginosus、Streptococcus mitisi、Streptococcus sanguinis)、Enterococcus faecalis*

歯内療法に関連するバイオフィルムの分類

根管内バイオフィルム	感染根管内象牙質で形成されたもの。
根尖孔外バイオフィルム	感染根管の根尖付近の歯根表面(セメント質)に形成されたもの。
根尖周囲バイオフィルム	感染根管の根尖病変内で形成されたもの。
生体材料周囲の感染	人工の生体材料表面に細菌が付着することで形成されたもの。

解説者コメント：NarayananとVaishnaviは、2010年の総説において歯内療法で観察される細菌とバイオフィルムを、上記の表のように分類して報告している。

13 細菌関連物質

出典 Narayanan LL, Vaishnavi C. Endodontic microbiology. J Conserv Dent 2010；13(4)：233-239.

細菌関連物質

LPS（リポ多糖）	グラム陰性菌の細胞壁表層を構成する内毒素。歯髄炎、根尖部の炎症、および根尖周囲の歯槽骨の吸収に関与する。
PG（ペプチドグリカン）	グラム陽性菌細胞壁の構成要素。自然免疫応答に関与するだけでなく、炎症促進性サイトカインや抗炎症性サイトカインの上方制御に関与する。
LTA（リポタイコ酸）	グラム陽性菌細胞壁の構成要素。LPSと類似した病原特性がある。細胞融解により放出後、標的細胞に結合すると、補体カスケードを活性化して損傷を引き起こす。
Fimbriae（繊毛）	多くのグラム陰性菌の表層に存在し、他の細菌と接着し、相互作用を生ずる。
Capsules（莢膜）	細菌細胞壁外層の層状の構造物。莢膜を有する菌はマクロファージによる貪食に抵抗する。
Extracellular vesicles（細胞外小胞）	グラム陰性菌より産生される。
Exotoxins（外毒素）	生細胞により産生される毒素。T細胞に過度な活性化や異常活性を引き起こす。
細胞外タンパク	細菌が産生する酵素であり、これらの酵素は細胞の融解時に放出され、細胞融解に働く。
Short-chain fatty acids（短鎖脂肪酸）	偏性嫌気性菌の発酵過程において産生される。炎症反応や炎症性サイトカイン放出の促進を助ける。
Polyamines（ポリアミン）	ポリカチオン分子であり、痛みに関連する臨床症状を引き起こす。
Superoxide anions（超酸化物）	赤血球の融解を引き起こす。

解説者コメント：根尖性歯周炎には、細菌だけでなく、上記の表のような細菌関連物質が関与していることをNarayananとVaishnavi(2010)は、報告している。

講演や雑誌でよく見る、あの分類および文献

14 幹細胞のタンパクおよび遺伝子のプロフィール

出典 Shi S, Bartold PM, Miura M, Seo BM, Robey PG, Gronthos S. The efficacy of mesenchymal stem cells to regenerate and repair dental structures. Orthod Craniofac Res 2005；8（3）：191-199.

口腔に関連した間葉系幹細胞のタンパクおよび遺伝子発現プロフィール

抗原	歯髄幹細胞	脱落乳歯歯髄幹細胞	歯根膜幹細胞	歯髄関連幹細胞
CD14	-	-	-	-
CD34	-	-	-	-
CD44	++	++	++	++
CD45	-	-	-	-
CD106	+	+/-	+/-	++
CD146	++/+/-	++/+/-	++/+/-	++/+/-
3G5	+/-	+/-	+/-	+/-
STRO-1	++/+/-	++/+/-	++/+/-	++/+/-
χ-SM actin	++/-	++/-	++/-	++/+/-
Collagen Type-I	++	++	++	++
Collagen Type-III	++/+	++/+/-	++/+/-	++/+
Alkaline phosphatase	++/+/-	++/+/-	++/+/-	++/+/-
Osteocalcin	++/+	++/+/-	++/-	+/-
Osteonectin	++/+	++/+	++/+	++/+
Osteopontin	+/-	+/-	+/-	+/-
Bone sialoprotein				
Scleraxis	+	+	++	+
Dentin sialophosphoprotein	-	-	-	-

(++)：強発現、(+)：弱発現、(-)：陰性、(/)：亜集団

解説者コメント：口腔に関連する間葉系幹細胞のタンパク発現や遺伝子発現プロフィールを表に示した。

クインテッセンス出版の書籍・雑誌は、歯学書専用通販サイト『歯学書.COM』にてご購入いただけます。

PCからのアクセスは…
歯学書 検索

携帯電話からのアクセスは…
QRコードからモバイルサイトへ

エンドのための重要20キーワードベスト240論文
世界のインパクトファクターを決めるトムソン・ロイター社が選出
――――――――――――――――――――――――――――――――
2015年11月10日　第1版第1刷発行

監　修	須田　英明（すだ ひであき）
著　者	金子　友厚（かねこ ともあつ）／伊藤　崇史（いとう たかふみ）／山本　信一（やまもと しんいち）
発　行　人	佐々木　一高
発　行　所	クインテッセンス出版株式会社 東京都文京区本郷3丁目2番6号　〒113-0033 クイントハウスビル　電話 (03)5842-2270(代表) 　　　　　　　　　　　　(03)5842-2272(営業部) 　　　　　　　　　　　　(03)5842-2275(the Quintessence編集部直通) web page address　http://www.quint-j.co.jp/
印刷・製本	横山印刷株式会社

――――――――――――――――――――――――――――――――
©2015　クインテッセンス出版株式会社　　禁無断転載・複写
Printed in Japan　　　　　　　　　　　落丁本・乱丁本はお取り替えします
　　　　　　　　　　　　　　　　　　　ISBN978-4-7812-0464-2　C3047

定価はカバーに表示してあります